Atlas of
CARDIOMETABOLIC RISK

Atlas of
CARDIOMETABOLIC RISK

William T Cefalu MD

Professor and Chief, Division of Nutrition and Chronic Diseases
Pennington Biomedical Research Center
Louisiana State University System
Baton Rouge, Louisiana, USA

and

Christopher P Cannon MD

Senior Investigator, Thrombolysis in Myocardial Infarction (TIMI) Study Group
Cardiovascular Division, Brigham and Women's Hospital
Associate Professor of Medicine, Harvard Medical School
Boston, Massachusetts, USA

Foreword by

Eugene Braunwald MD

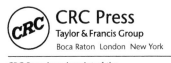

CRC Press
Taylor & Francis Group
Boca Raton London New York

CRC Press is an imprint of the
Taylor & Francis Group, an **informa** business

CRC Press
Taylor & Francis Group
6000 Broken Sound Parkway NW, Suite 300
Boca Raton, FL 33487-2742

First issued in paperback 2019

© 2007 by Taylor & Francis Group, LLC
CRC Press is an imprint of Taylor & Francis Group, an Informa business

No claim to original U.S. Government works

ISBN-13: 978-0-8493-7053-3 (hbk)
ISBN-13: 978-0-367-38924-6 (pbk)

Cover illustrations courtesy of: GA Bray, GBM Lindop, IN Scobie, PF Semple and HC Stary

Visit the Taylor & Francis Web site at
http://www.taylorandfrancis.com

and the CRC Press Web site at

Foreword

At the beginning of the twentieth century cardiovascular disease was responsible for approximately 10% of all deaths in the United States. During the first half of the century, with urbanization and the transition from a largely agricultural to an industrial economy, the percentage of deaths due to cardiovascular disease rose rapidly to about 35%, becoming the most common cause of mortality in the United States and, indeed, in the entire industrialized world. By mid-century, the recognition that an acute coronary event is not "a bolt out of the blue" but often occurs in susceptible patients in whom the classic coronary risk factors of hypercholesterolemia, hypertension, and/or smoking had been present sparked an interest in preventive measures. The development of coronary care units, coronary revascularization, as well as antihypertensive and cholesterol-reducing agents first stopped the steady rise in cardiovascular deaths and then delayed such deaths substantially. By the beginning of the last decade of the century it appeared that the tide had turned and that, at last, atherosclerotic vascular disease was beginning to come under control.

However, despite this encouraging progress, all was not well. With the transition from the industrial economy to an information-service economy, the wide availability and popularity of very high caloric, fast foods (the "McDonald's culture") and the reduction in physical activity, the twin epidemics of type 2 diabetes and obesity began to grow at an alarming rate. The percentage of the population that is overweight or obese has risen by 5% per decade since 1960, and the percentage with diabetes has almost doubled in just the last ten years. A cluster of risk factors, including but not limited to insulin resistance, central obesity, dyslipidemia, impaired glucose tolerance, essential hypertension and inflammation is associated with a state of increased cardiometabolic risk that is now present in at least one quarter of the adult population. As we approach the end of the first decade of the twenty-first century, the seeming relentless rise in cardiometabolic risk threatens to reverse the earlier progress in the battle against atherosclerotic coronary and non-coronary vascular disease.

In order to control cardiometabolic risk we must first understand this cluster of risk factors and examine the several modes of prevention and treatment that are now or will soon be at our disposal. Dr Cefalu, an expert on metabolic diseases, and Dr Cannon, a cardiologist, have teamed up with a group of talented authors to prepare this splendid *Atlas of Cardiometabolic Risk*. The excellent explanatory diagrams and the lucid accompanying text provide the reader with the knowledge required to engage in this next critical battle against atherosclerotic cardiovascular disease.

Eugene Braunwald, MD
Brigham and Women's Hospital
Harvard Medical School
Boston, MA

Preface

Cardiovascular disease is the leading cause of death and disability worldwide. Although our understanding of this disease has progressed enormously, we have much to improve in identification of the disease and applying optimal treatments to prevent progression of disease and its consequences.

Beginning nearly 50 years ago, the Framingham Heart Study forever changed our approach to coronary artery disease by identifying major risk factors for myocardial infarction (MI) – namely hypertension, smoking, hypercholesterolemia, diabetes and a family history of MI. Since then, countless other risk factors and markers of disease have been identified. Our current approach to prevention (either primary prevention of a first event, or secondary prevention of recurrent events) is largely focused on controlling these individual risk factors. This single risk factor approach has led to multiple classes of drugs to treat each condition, and guidelines are developed centered on improvements of each one (e.g., hypertension – JNC VII, or the ADA) In addition, decades ago, the United States government established national programs, such as the National Cholesterol Education Program (NCEP) that develops guidelines for management of cholesterol.

A new approach is emerging however – that looks not at individual risk factors, but at the overall risk of disease in a patient. This involves looking at a long list of contributing risk factors – to assess a patient's overall cardiometabolic risk. It is this new approach to diagnosis and management that this book embraces. We aim to provide the best possible care to our patients, and taking this comprehensive approach is the best strategy to do so.

We cover many aspects of cardiometabolic risk in this Atlas. The initial chapters delve into the new understanding of the pathophysiology of the cardiometabolic risk, with colorful illustrations of the various pathways involved. Then, we cover many of the markers of cardiometabolic risk that can be used to identify patients in clinical practice. The final chapters review the newest trial data on the natural history of the disease with clinical outcomes of patients, as well as a brief overview of all the current treatments for cardiometabolic risk. We hope that this book will provide clinicians with a readily accessible guide to this important disease, that will help in caring for this large group of patients.

Christopher P Cannon, MD
William T Cefalu, MD

Contents

Contributors

Christopher P Cannon MD
TIMI Study Group
Cardiovascular Division
Department of Medicine
Brigham and Women's Hospital
Harvard Medical School, Boston, MA, USA

William T Cefalu MD
Division of Nutrition and Chronic Diseases
Pennington Biomedical Research Center
Louisiana State University System
Baton Rouge, LA, USA

Gregory Piazza MD
Division of Cardiology
Department of Medicine
Beth Israel Deaconess Medical Center
Harvard Medical School
Boston, MA, USA

Kausik K Ray MD
Department of Public Health and Primary Care
University of Cambridge
and
Addenbrooke's Hospital
Cambridge, UK

Benjamin A Steinberg BA
Department of Medicine
Brigham and Women's Hospital
Harvard Medical School, Boston, MA, USA

1 Classification and evolution of increased cardiometabolic risk states

It has been accurately observed that certain risk factors in humans appear to 'cluster' with clinical states such as obesity and type 2 diabetes. Specifically, this risk factor clustering, and the association with insulin resistance, led investigators to propose the existence of a unique pathophysiological condition[1]. Many names have been provided to describe this clinical state including 'metabolic syndrome', 'syndrome X', and 'insulin resistance syndrome'[1]. The particular names that refer to this risk factor clustering describe the human condition characterized by the presence of co-existing traditional risk factors for cardiovascular disease (CVD), such as hypertension, dyslipidemia, glucose intolerance, obesity, and insulin resistance, in addition to non-traditional CVD risk factors, such as inflammatory processes and abnormalities of the blood coagulation system[2-6]. Table 1.1 lists conditions and components associated with the clustering of risk factors. As seen, the components that are associated with risk factor clustering, e.g. 'metabolic syndrome', include not only many of the traditional risk factors, e.g. lipids, obesity, hypertension, but also components that represent aspects of vascular health, such as endothelial dysfunction, inflammation, and parameters assessing blood coagulability[7]. Recently, a joint statement released by the American Diabetes Association (ADA) suggested that, as a construct that denoted risk factor clustering, 'metabolic syndrome' has been a useful paradigm in that it draws attention to the fact that risk factors tend to cluster in patients[1]. However, the ADA felt that, while there is no doubt that certain CVD risk factors cluster, it was their impression that metabolic syndrome has

Table 1.1 Proposed components and associated findings felt to represent metabolic syndrome. The components listed represent not only many of the traditional risk factors, e.g. lipids, obesity, hypertension, but also components that represent aspects of vascular health such as endothelial dysfunction. In addition, parameters assessing inflammation, blood coagulability and insulin resistance are included. From reference 7, with permission

1. Insulin resistance*
2. Hyperinsulinemia*
3. Obesity: visceral (central), but also generalized obesity*
4. Dyslipidemia: high triglycerides, low HDL, small dense LDL*
5. Adipocyte dysfunction
6. Impaired glucose tolerance or type 2 diabetes mellitus*
7. Fatty liver (non-alcoholic steatohepatosis, steatohepatitis)
8. Essential hypertension: increased systolic and diastolic blood pressure
9. Endothelial dysfunction
10. Renal dysfunction: micro- or macroalbuminuria
11. Polycystic ovary syndrome
12. Inflammation: increased CRP and other inflammatory markers
13. Hypercoagulability: increased fibrinogen and PAI-1
14. Atherosclerosis leading to increased cardiovascular morbidity and mortality*

* Most widely incorporated into the definition of metabolic syndrome
CRP, C-reactive protein; PAI-1, plasminogen activator inhibitor type 1

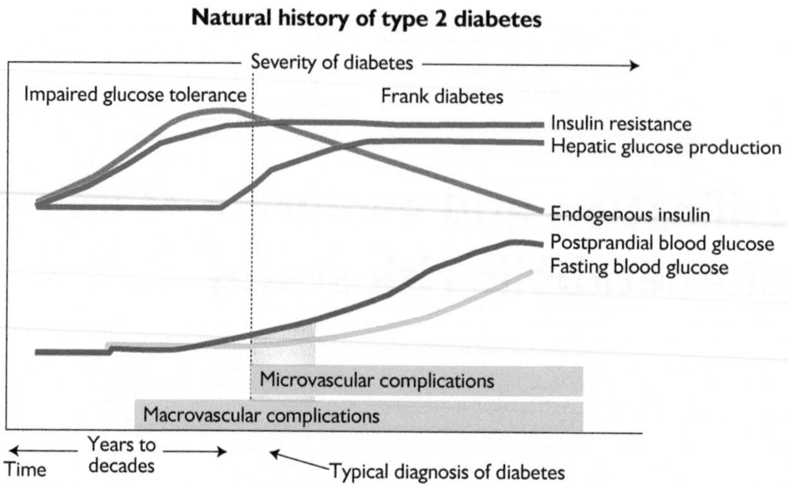

Natural history of type 2 diabetes

Figure 1.1 Schematic demonstrating where the presence of metabolic syndrome fits into the natural history of type 2 diabetes. Prior to the development of clinical overt hyperglycemia and the diagnosis of type 2 diabetes, it is observed that insulin resistance may develop in the majority of individuals, primarily associated with obesity. The development of insulin resistance in an individual will need to be compensated by hyperinsulinemia in order to maintain normal glucose tolerance. However, when the insulin secretory capacity of the β cell begins to diminish such that the pancreatic function now fails to compensate for the insulin resistance, a state of relative 'insulin deficiency' leading to hyperglycemia is observed. It is at this stage that impaired glucose tolerance and impaired fasting glucose may be present. With worsening pancreatic dysfunction and the inability to compensate fully for the degree of insulin resistance, hyperglycemia continues to increase and clinically overt type 2 diabetes develops. Adapted from reference 9, with permission

been imprecisely defined[1]. For purpose of this Atlas, we will refer to the clustering of CVD risk factors as indicative of a state of increased cardiometabolic risk.

Whereas the etiology of cardiometabolic risk is not specifically known, it is well established that obesity and insulin resistance are generally present[2–4]. Insulin resistance, defined as a clinical state in which a normal or elevated insulin level produces an impaired biological response, is considered to be a hallmark for the presence of metabolic syndrome. Insulin resistance can be secondary to rare conditions such as abnormal insulin molecules, circulating insulin antagonists (e.g. glucocorticoids, growth hormone, anti-insulin antibodies), or even secondary to genetic syndromes such as the muscular dystrophies[8]. However, the insulin resistance considered as part of the metabolic syndrome essentially represents a target-tissue (i.e. skeletal muscle) defect in insulin action and accounts for the overwhelming majority of cases of insulin resistance reported for the human condition[8]. The cellular mechanisms that contribute to insulin resistance are not

fully understood, but will be discussed in more detail in Chapter 2.

The risk factor clustering that defines the state of increased cardiometabolic risk contributes greatly to increased morbidity and mortality in humans on several levels. First, these risk factors are present at the 'pre-diabetic' state. Specifically, and as demonstrated in Figure 1.1, it is now well accepted that the presence of insulin resistance in an individual will need to be compensated by hyperinsulinemia in order to maintain normal glucose tolerance[10–14]. It is also observed that in those individuals who develop diabetes, a progressive loss of the insulin secretory capacity of β-cells appears to begin years before the clinical diagnosis of diabetes. The pancreatic dysfunction fails to compensate for the insulin resistance and results in a state of relative 'insulin deficiency' leading to hyperglycemia. It is at this stage that impaired glucose tolerance and impaired fasting glucose may be present. With worsening pancreatic dysfunction and the inability to compensate fully for the degree of insulin resistance, hyperglycemia continues to increase and

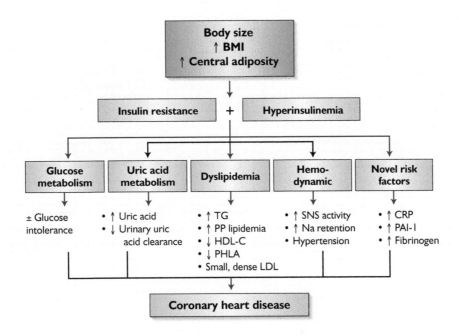

Figure 1.2 The current perspective on the relationship between metabolic syndrome and coronary heart disease. The presence of obesity in an individual is highly associated with the development of insulin resistance and hyperinsulinemia. Many traditional risk factors for CVD are related to the development of metabolic syndrome and these include glucose abnormalities, dyslipidemia and hemodynamic factors. However, novel risk factors such as abnormalities in inflammatory markers, i.e. C-reactive protein (CRP) and coagulopathy (plasminogen activator inhibitor-1 (PAI-1)) also appear to play a role. BMI, body mass index; HDL-C, high-density lipoprotein cholesterol; LDL, low-density lipoprotein; PHLA, postheparin lipolytic activity; PP, postprandial; SNS, sympathetic nervous system; TG, triglycerides. These factors are highly related to the development of coronary heart disease. From reference 17, with permission

clinically overt type 2 diabetes becomes present (Figure 1.1). Thus, the CVD risk factor clustering and the associated insulin resistance confers an increased cardiometabolic risk state and figures prominently in the natural history of type 2 diabetes (Figure 1.1).

A second major reason why a state of increased cardiometabolic risk contributes to increased morbidity and mortality in humans is the association with cardiovascular disease[6,15,16]. Coexisting cardiovascular risk factors, such as dyslipidemia, hypertension, inflammatory markers, and coagulopathy, are highly associated with the 'pre-diabetic' state as defined by obesity and insulin resistance, and have been defined in the past as components of the metabolic syndrome (Table 1.1). Therefore, as demonstrated, the presence of insulin resistance and obesity in 'pre-diabetes' will be associated with increasing prevalence of the CVD risk factors (Figure 1.2). Each risk factor, when considered alone, increases CVD risk but, more

importantly, in combination they provide a 'synergistic' or 'additive' effect (Figure 1.3). For example, Lakka and his research team used definitions of metabolic syndrome by criteria as established by the National Cholesterol Education Program (NCEP) and the World Health Organization (WHO), and evaluated relative risk of death from coronary heart disease (CHD) during an 11-year follow-up in 1209 middle-aged men[19]. After correcting for multiple factors, the presence of the metabolic syndrome resulted in a 2.5–4-fold increase in relative risk for CVD death regardless of the criteria used (Figure 1.4). With the understanding that metabolic syndrome may precede the development of diabetes by many years (see Figure 1.1), the presence of this condition may partially explain the increase in CVD risk observed years before the diagnosis of diabetes, as outlined in Figures 1.5 and 1.6. Specifically, Hu *et al.* reported that the relative risk for CVD was significantly increased beginning as early

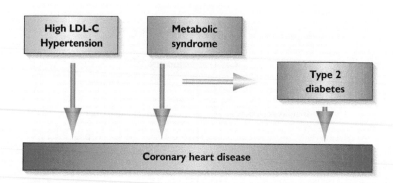

Figure 1.3 The presence of individual cardiovascular disease risk factors (hypertension, dyslipidemia) is clearly related to the development of coronary heart disease. However, when many of these factors are present in the same individual (such as individuals with metabolic syndrome), an 'additive' or 'synergistic' effect may be observed. LDL-C, low-density lipoprotein cholesterol. Adapted from reference 18

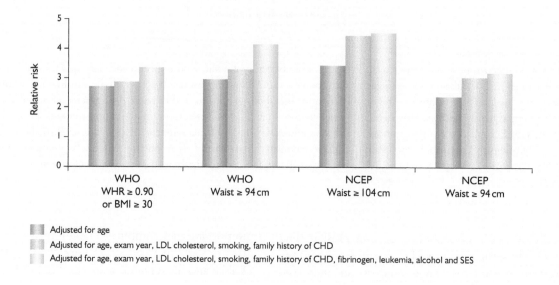

Figure 1.4 Relative risk of death from coronary heart disease (CHD) for metabolic syndrome during an 11-year follow-up of 1209 middle-aged men. As observed, regardless of whether the criteria as established for metabolic syndrome for the World Health Organization (WHO) or National Cholesterol Education Program (NCEP) were used, individuals with central obesity had an increased relative risk for CHD. In addition, these observations persisted regardless of the various statistical adjustments for lipids, smoking, family history, and other socioeconomic factors. BMI, body mass index; LDL, low-density lipoprotein; SES, socioeconomic status; WHR, waist-to-hip ratio. Adapted from reference 19

as 15 years before the diagnosis of diabetes, and the CVD risk increased significantly in the years closer to the actual time the clinical diagnosis of diabetes was made (Figure 1.5)[20]. Thus, the current perspective of increase in cardiometabolic risk as it relates to development of coronary heart disease is outlined schematically in Figure 1.6. The relationship of risk factors to CVD will be covered in more detail in later chapters.

In the past, a number of criteria have been suggested to meet those for being classified as having 'metabolic syndrome' for any given individual. For example, Table 1.2 outlines the criteria as previously suggested by the National Cholesterol Education Program (NCEP-ATP III)[18]. Although ATP III did not make any single risk factor (e.g. abdominal obesity) a requirement for diagnosis, it nonetheless espoused the

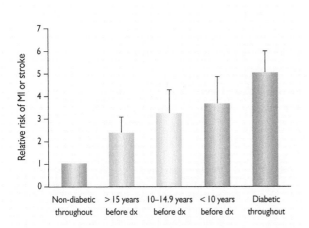

Figure 1.5 Relative risk of myocardial infarction (MI) or stroke in pre-diabetes. Hu and his collaborators, from the Nurses' Health Study, reported that the relative risk for cardiovascular disease (CVD) was significantly increased beginning as early as 15 years before the diagnosis (dx) of diabetes, and the CVD risk increased significantly in the years closer to the actual time the clinical diagnosis of diabetes was made. Adapted from reference 20, reproduced with permission

position that abdominal obesity is an important underlying risk factor for the syndrome. Abdominal obesity at these cut-off points (see Table 1.2) was not made a prerequisite for diagnosis because lesser degrees of abdominal girth often associate with other ATP III criteria. In fact, some individuals or ethnic groups (e.g. Asians, especially South Asians) appear to be susceptible to development of the metabolic syndrome at waist circumferences below ATP III cut-off points. Thus, ATP III specifically noted that some individuals having only two other metabolic syndrome criteria appear to be insulin resistant even when the waist circumference is only marginally elevated, e.g. 94–101 cm in men or 80–87 cm in women. The WHO had very similar criteria as outlined in Table 1.3. However, required criteria for WHO guidelines include the presence of impaired glucose tolerance (IGT), impaired fasting glucose (IFG), diabetes, or insulin resistance. The American Association of Clinical Endocrinologists (AACE) have also provided guidelines based on clinical signs, and these are compared with both the NCEP and WHO criteria (Table 1.4). In 2003, the AACE modified ATP III criteria to refocus

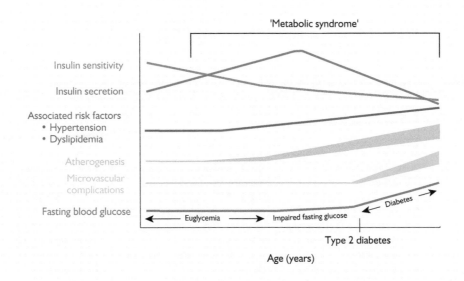

Figure 1.6 Schematic demonstrating the development of metabolic syndrome in the natural history of type 2 diabetes. As shown, with the development of metabolic syndrome, there is an increasing prevalence of the associated risk factors that are observed many years before the diagnosis of type 2 diabetes is made. In addition, the CVD risk is greatly accelerated during this time. Therefore, CVD risk is elevated many years prior to the diagnosis of diabetes in large part owing to the presence of metabolic syndrome. When the pancreas fails to compensate for the insulin resistance, hyperglycemia ensues, which also contributes greatly to CVD risk. From reference 14, with permission

on insulin resistance as the primary cause of metabolic risk factors[23]. Major criteria included were glucose levels indicative of impaired glucose tolerance, elevated triglycerides, reduced HDL cholesterol, elevated blood pressure, and obesity. No specified number of factors qualified for diagnosis, which was left to clinical judgment.

In April of 2005, the International Diabetes Federation (IDF) presented a new consensus definition that is an important modification of the previously used ATP III definition[24]. The IDF definition clearly outlined the complexity of the syndrome and also suggested that central obesity should be a prerequisite for the syndrome. More importantly, the IDF

Table 1.2 Diagnosis of metabolic syndrome as suggested by the National Cholesterol Education Program. As outlined, diagnosis is established when ≥ 3 of these risk factors are present. From reference 18, with permission

Risk factor	Defining level
Abdominal obesity* (waist circumference†)	
Men	> 102 cm (> 40 in)
Women	> 88 cm (> 35 in)
TG	≥ 150 mg/dL
HDL-C	
Men	< 40 mg/dL
Women	< 50 mg/dL
Blood pressure	≥ 130/≥ 85 mmHg
Fasting glucose	≥ 110 mg/dL

HDL-C, high-density lipoprotein cholesterol; TG, triglycerides
*Abdominal obesity is more highly correlated with metabolic risk factors than is increased body mass index
†Some men develop metabolic risk factors when the circumference is only marginally increased

Table 1.3 The World Health Organization (WHO) definition of metabolic syndrome*. As outlined, the parameters appear similar to the National Cholesterol Education Program ATP III criteria. However, WHO criteria would include measures of insulin resistance, if these are available in a particular subject

Impaired glucose tolerance, impaired fasting glucose, diabetes and/or insulin resistance	
And ≥ 2 of the following:	
Abdominal obesity	
BMI	> 30 kg/m² or
Waist-to-hip ratio	> 0.85 women
	> 0.90 men
Dyslipidemia	
Triglycerides	≥ 150 mg/dL or
HDL	< 35 mg/dL in men
	< 39 mg/dL women
Blood pressure	≥ 140/90 mmHg
Microalbuminuria	
Urinary excretion rate	≥ 20 µg/min or
Albumin–creatinine ratio	≥ 20 mg/g

*WHO Definition, Diagnosis and Classification of Diabetes and its Complications. Report of WHO Consultation. Geneva: WHO, 1999
BMI, body mass index; HDL, high-density lipoprotein

Table 1.4 A comparison of the specific criteria necessary for the definition of metabolic syndrome from the American Diabetes Association (ADA), National Cholesterol Education Program (NCEP), World Health Organization (WHO), and the American Association of Clinical Endocrinologists (AACE). From reference 7, with permission

ADA	NCEP*	WHO†	AACE‡
Glucose intolerance	Fasting plasma glucose 110–125 mg/dL	Type 2 diabetes, impaired glucose tolerance, or insulin resistance by HOMA-IR	Fasting plasma glucose 110–125 mg/dL or 2-h post-75 g glucose challenge > 140 mg/dL
Central obesity	Waist circumference > 40 in (men) or > 35 in (women)	BMI > 30 or waist-to-hip ratio > 0.90 (men) or > 0.85 (women)	BMI ≥ 25 or waist circumference > 40 in (men) or > 35 in (women)
Dyslipidemia: high TG, low HDL, small dense LDL	TG ≥ 150 mg/dL, HDL < 40 (men), HDL < 50 (women)	TG ≥ 150 mg/dL, HDL < 35 (men), HDL < 39 (women)	TG ≥ 150 mg/dL, HDL < 40 (men), HDL < 50 (women)
Hypertension	Blood pressure ≥ 130/85 mmHg	On medication or untreated blood pressure ≥ 140/90 mmHg	High blood pressure ≥ 130/85 mmHg
		Microalbuminuria > 20 µg/min	

*NCEP: must meet 3 of 5 criteria (low HDL and high triglycerides are 2 criteria)
†WHO: must meet glucose/insulin criterion and 2 more
‡AACE: these key clinical signs are considered risk factors. Other risk factors include: polycystic ovary syndrome; sedentary lifestyle; age; ethnicity (certain groups); and family history of type 2 diabetes, hypertension, or cardiovascular disease
BMI, body mass index; HDL, high-density lipoprotein; HOMA-IR, homeostasis model assessment; LDL, low-density lipoprotein; TG, triglycerides

definition attempted to provide a more appropriate definition for abdominal obesity. When such is present, two additional factors originally listed in the ATP III definition are sufficient for diagnosis. The IDF recognized and emphasized ethnic differences in the correlation between abdominal obesity and other metabolic syndrome risk factors. For this reason, criteria of abdominal obesity were specified by nationality or ethnicity based on best available population estimates. The most recent American Heart Association/National Heart, Lung, and Blood Institute (AHA/NHLBI) statement, in contrast to IDF, maintains the ATP III criteria except for minor modifications (Table 1.5)[25]. They suggested lowering of the threshold previously set for impaired fasting glucose to 100 mg/dL and they did not adjust the existing US waist circumference cri-

teria. Depending on the definition, it has been estimated that one in four adults may have either diabetes or the metabolic syndrome (Figure 1.7)[26].

Given the CVD significance of the clustering of risk factors, the fact that a state of increased cardiometabolic risk may be three to four times as common as diabetes, and the observation that obesity and other risk factors (i.e. dyslipidemia and diabetes) have become global health epidemics, a state of increased cardiometabolic risk represents a serious public health concern. Currently, it is estimated that approximately 7–8% of the population in the USA suffer from the complications of adult-onset diabetes[27]. However, the prevalence of diabetes in the USA has increased dramatically over the recent past. Figure 1.8 demonstrates the estimated prevalence of diabetes as established for the USA in the year 1990, where an estimated prevalence was 4.9%, compared with the data as obtained in the year 2001 with an estimated prevalence of 7.9%[28].

In large part, the increase in diabetes appears to be secondary to the increase in obesity. Clearly, there is no question that the US population has had a significant increase in obesity over the past 40 years. Figure 1.9 demonstrates the percentage of the population since 1960 that are now classified as either obese or overweight. As shown, there has been a steady increase in individuals classified as obese[29]. Since 1990, however, the prevalence of obesity has increased by 61%[30–32]. As seen in Figure 1.10, the increasing prevalence of

Table 1.5 Criteria for clinical diagnosis of metabolic syndrome. From reference 25, with permission

Measure (any 3 of 5 constitute diagnosis of metabolic syndrome)	Categorical cut-off points
Elevated waist circumference*†	≥ 102 cm (≥ 40 inches) in men ≥ 88 cm (≥ 35 inches) in women
Elevated triglycerides	≥ 150 mg/dL (1.7 mmol/L) or On drug treatment for elevated triglycerides‡
Reduced HDL-C	< 40 mg/dL (1.03 mmol/L) in men < 50 mg/dL (1.3 mmol/L) in women or On drug treatment for reduced HDL-C‡
Elevated blood pressure	≥ 130 mmHg systolic blood pressure or ≥ 85 mmHg diastolic blood pressure or On antihypertensive drug treatment in a patient with a history of hypertension
Elevated fasting glucose	≥ 100 mg/dL or On drug treatment for elevated glucose

*To measure waist circumference, locate top of right iliac crest. Place a measuring tape in a horizontal plane around abdomen at level of iliac crest. Before reading tape measure, ensure that tape is snug but does not compress the skin and is parallel to floor. Measurement is made at the end of a normal expiration
†Some US adults of non-Asian origin (e.g. white, black, Hispanic) with marginally increased waist circumference (e.g. 94–101 cm (37–39 inches) in men and 80–87 cm (31–34 inches) in women) may have strong genetic contribution to insulin resistance and should benefit from changes in lifestyle habits, similar to men with categorical increases in waist circumference. Lower waist circumference cutpoint (e.g. ≥ 90 cm (35 inches) in men and ≥ 80 cm (31 inches) in women) appears to be appropriate for Asian Americans
‡Fibrates and nicotinic acid are the most commonly used drugs for elevated triglyceride (TG) and reduced high-density lipoprotein cholesterol(HDL-C). Patients taking one of these drugs are presumed to have high TG and low HDL

Table 1.6 Diabetes has become a worldwide health concern. As observed, there appears to be no area of the world that has not observed a tremendous rise in new cases of diabetes. On current estimates, approximately 360 million people worldwide will have diabetes by the year 2030. From reference 21, with permission

Ranking	2000		2030	
	Country	People with diabetes (millions)	Country	People with diabetes (millions)
1	India	31.7	India	79.4
2	China	20.8	China	42.3
3	USA	17.7	USA	30.3
4	Indonesia	8.4	Indonesia	21.3
5	Japan	6.8	Pakistan	13.9
6	Pakistan	5.2	Brazil	11.3
7	Russian Federation	4.6	Bangladesh	11.1
8	Brazil	4.6	Japan	8.9
9	Italy	4.3	Philippines	7.8
10	Bangladesh	3.2	Egypt	6.7

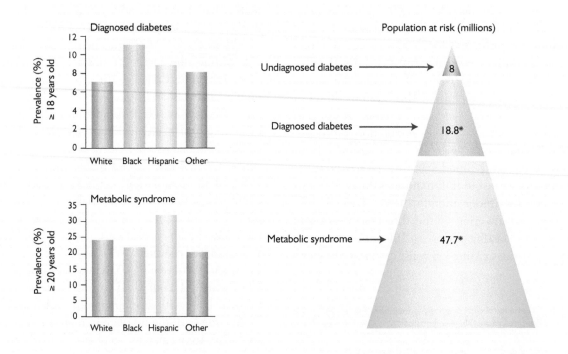

Figure 1.7 Schematic representing prevalence of metabolic syndrome. Estimates have suggested that over 18 million individuals residing in the USA have diabetes, with significant numbers undiagnosed. Depending on the criteria used, it is estimated that one in four adults may have diabetes or the metabolic syndrome. From references 26 and 28, with permission

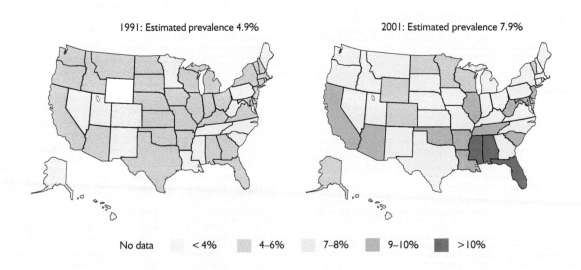

Figure 1.8 Estimated prevalence of diabetes in the USA in 1991 and 2001 based on a telephone survey of 195 005 adults aged 18 or over. As shown, several states had higher prevalence of diabetes in 1990, many > 7%. As also shown, by the year 2001, most of the other states had observed an increase in prevalence of > 7%, with the increase being much higher in many states. From reference 28, with permission

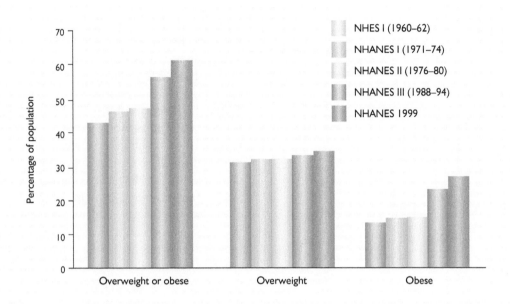

Figure 1.9 The increase in numbers of individuals classified as being overweight or obese since 1960. As clearly shown, the percentage of the US population classified as obese has increased dramatically. NHES, National Health Examination Survey; NHANES, National Health and Nutrition Examination Survey. From reference 29, with permission

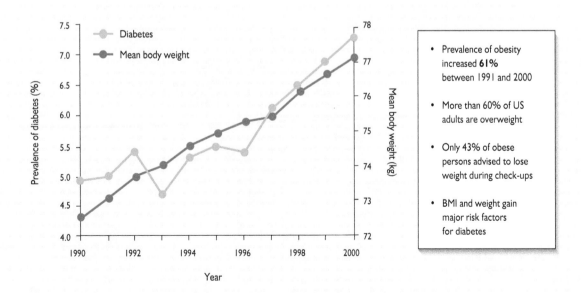

Figure 1.10 Prevalence of diabetes and obesity in the USA since 1990. As shown, the increase in diabetes prevalence appears to mirror the increase in rates of obesity. It is observed that the prevalence of obesity increased by 61% from 1991 to 2000. These observations support the well-observed concept that weight gain is a major risk factor for diabetes. BMI, body mass index. Compiled from references 30, 31 and 32, with permission

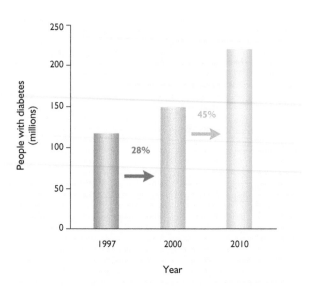

Figure 1.11 Estimated number of individuals with type 2 diabetes who are expected to have diabetes by the year 2010. This would represent a 45% increase since the year 2000. Adapted from reference 33

diabetes appears to mirror closely the increasing prevalence of obesity. However, despite the findings of obesity and diabetes in the USA, this is truly a global problem. Based on the estimated number of people with diabetes, it is projected that by the year 2010, there will be 221 million people worldwide with diabetes (Figure 1.11) and 360 million by the year 2030 (Table 1.6). As is outlined in Figure 1.12, it is clear that very few areas of the world are immune to developing diabetes. The major concern with the epidemic of diabetes will be the development of the devastating complications of diabetes as outlined in Figure 1.13. With specific reference to metabolic syndrome, it is clear that the obesity epidemic contributes greatly to the presence of metabolic syndrome and that the prevalence of the metabolic syndrome increases with age. It is estimated that, by the time individuals reach the age of 60 years, approximately 40% may have the metabolic syndrome (Figure 1.14)[26]. Minority ethnic groups are at even greater risk. Therefore, it is not surprising that the WHO considers it to be one of the top ten most dangerous diseases in the world today[35,36].

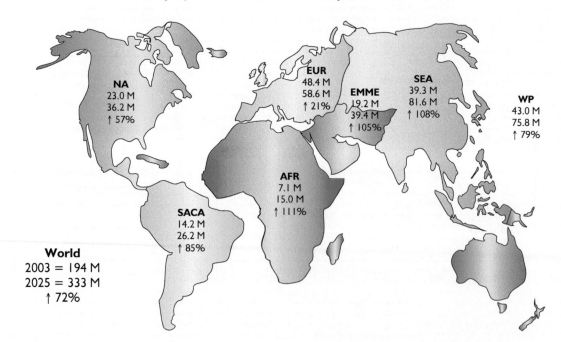

Figure 1.12 Global projections for the diabetes epidemic. As shown, an increase in new cases of diabetes will be observed in all parts of the world. From reference 34, with permission

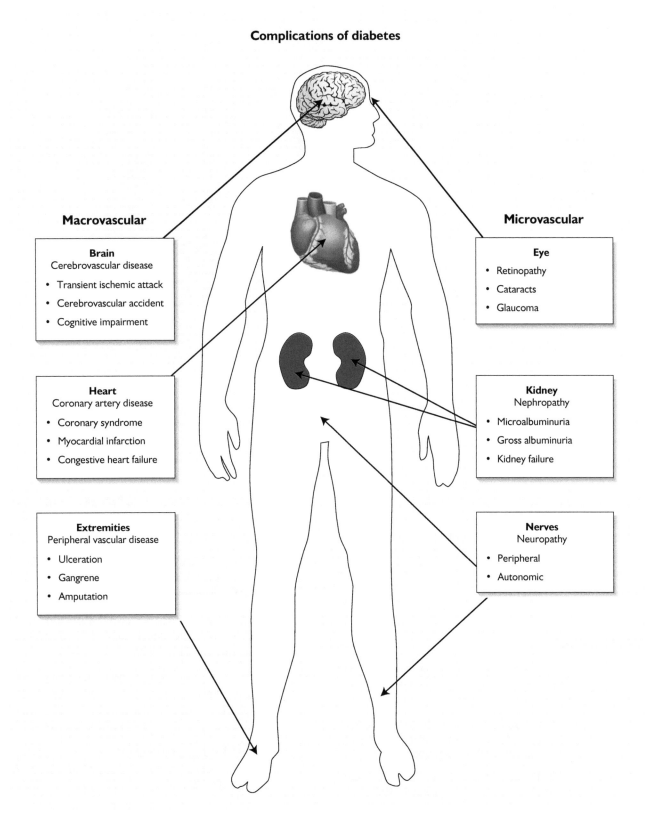

Figure 1.13   Schematic demonstrating micro- and macrovascular complications of diabetes

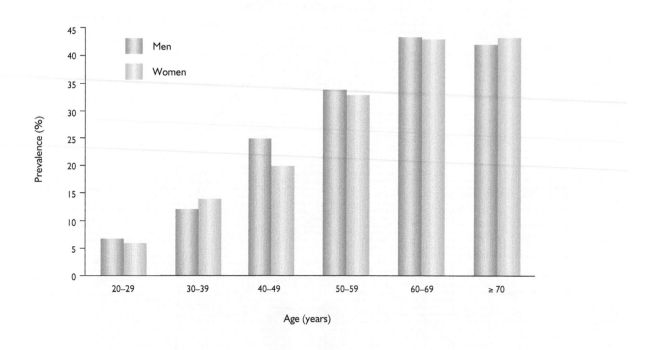

Figure 1.14 Metabolic syndrome prevalence among US adults. Clearly there is increasing prevalence in older individuals such that, by age 60, over 40% of the population may have criteria for metabolic syndrome. From reference 26, with permission

Successful strategies to intervene in the development of the 'metabolic syndrome' are urgently needed. Such interventions will be discussed in later chapters.

In summary, the development of metabolic syndrome is a threat to public health worldwide and is increasing at epidemic proportions.

REFERENCES

1. Kahn R, Buse J, Ferrannini E, Stern M. The metabolic syndrome: time for a critical appraisal. Diabetes Care 2005; 28: 2289–304

2. DeFronzo RA. Insulin resistance, hyperinsulinemia, and coronary artery disease: a complex metabolic web. J Cardiovasc Pharmacol 1992; 20 (Suppl 11): S1–16

3. Reaven GM. Banting lecture 1988. Role of insulin resistance in human disease. Diabetes 1988; 37: 1595–607

4. Haffner SM. The insulin resistance syndrome revisited. Diabetes Care 1996; 19: 275–7

5. Liese AD, Mayer-Davis EJ, Haffner SM. Development of the multiple metabolic syndrome: an epidemiologic perspective. Epidemiol Rev 1998; 20: 157–72

6. Isomaa B, Almgren P, Tuomi T, et al. Cardiovascular morbidity and mortality associated with the metabolic syndrome. Diabetes Care 2001; 24: 683–9

7. Miranda PJ, DeFronzo RA, Califf RM, Gryton JR. Metabolic syndrome: definition, pathophysiology and mechanisms. Am Heart J 2005; 149: 33–45

8. Hunter SJ, Garvey WT. Insulin action and insulin resistance: diseases involving defects in insulin receptors, signal transduction, and the glucose transport effector system. Am J Med 1998; 105: 331–45

9. Ramlo-Halsted BA, Edelman SV. The natural history of type 2 diabetes. Primary Care Clinics of North America 1999;26:771–89

10. Kahn SE. The importance of the beta-cell in the pathogenesis of type 2 diabetes. Am J Med 2000; 108 (Suppl 6a): 2S–8S

11. Buchanan TA. Pancreatic beta-cell loss and preservation in type 2 diabetes. Clin Ther 2003; 25 (Suppl B): B32–46

12. Weyer C, Bogardus C, Mott DM, Pratley RE. The natural history of insulin secretory dysfunction and insulin resistance in the pathogenesis of type 2 diabetes mellitus. J Clin Invest 1999; 104: 787–94

13. Weyer C, Tataranni PA, Bogardus C, Pratley RE. Insulin resistance and insulin secretory dysfunction are independent predictors of worsening of glucose tolerance during each stage of type 2 diabetes development. Diabetes Care 2001; 24: 89–94

14. Cefalu WT. Insulin resistance. In Leahy J, Clark N, Cefalu WT, eds. The Medical Management of Diabetes Mellitus. New York: Marcel Dekker, 2000: 57–75

15. McLaughlin T, Allison G, Abbasi F, et al. Prevalence of insulin resistance and associated cardiovascular disease risk factors among normal weight, overweight, and obese individuals. Metabolism 2004; 53: 495–9

16. Shirai K. Obesity as the core of the metabolic syndrome and the management of coronary heart disease. Curr Med Res Opin 2004; 20: 295–304

17. Reaven G. Syndrome X: 10 years after. Drugs 1999; 58 (Suppl 1): 19–20

18. Executive Summary of the Third Report of The National Cholesterol Education Program (NCEP). Expert Panel on Detection, Evaluation, and Treatment of High Blood Cholesterol in Adults (Adult Treatment Panel III). JAMA 2001; 285: 2486–97

19. Lakka HM, Laaksonen DE, Lakka TA, et al. The metabolic syndrome and total and cardiovascular disease mortality in middle-aged men. JAMA 2002; 288: 2709–16

20. Hu FB, Stampfer MJ, Haffner SM, et al. Elevated risk of cardiovascular disease prior to clinical diagnosis of type 2 diabetes. Diabetes Care 2002; 25: 1129–34

21. Wild S, Roglic G, Green A, et al. Global prevalence of diabetes: estimates for the year 2000 and projections for 2030. Diabetes Care 2004; 27: 1047–53

22. Alberti KG, Zimmet PZ. Definition, diagnosis and classification of diabetes mellitus and its complications. Part 1: diagnosis and classification of diabetes mellitus provisional report of a WHO consultation. Diabet Med 1998; 15: 539–53

23. Einhorn D, Reaven GM, Cobin RH, et al. American College of Endocrinology position statement on the insulin resistance syndrome. Endocr Pract 2003; 9: 237–52

24. Alberti KGMM, Zimmet P, Shaw J, for the IDF Epidemiology Task Force Consensus Group. The metabolic syndrome – a new world wide definition. Lancet 2005; 366: 1059–62

25. Grundy SM, Cleeman JI, Daniels SR, et al. Diagnosis and management of the metabolic syndrome: an American Heart Association/National Heart, Lung, and Blood Institute Scientific Statement. Circulation 2005; 112: 2735–52

26. Ford ES, Giles WH, Dietz WH. Prevalence of the metabolic syndrome among US adults: findings from the third National Health and Nutrition Examination Survey. JAMA 2002; 287: 356–9

27. Centers for Disease Control and Prevention (CDC). Diabetes prevalence among American Indians and Alaska Natives and the overall population – United States, 1994–2. MMWR Morb Mortal Wkly Rep 2003; 52: 702–4

28. Mokdad AH, Ford ES, Bowman BA, et al. Prevalence of obesity, diabetes, and obesity-related health risk factors, 2001. JAMA 2003; 289: 76–9

29. AGA Technical Review on Obesity. Gastroenterology 2002; 123: 882–932

30. Mokdad AH, Ford ES, Bowman RA, et al. Diabetes trends in the US: 1990–1998. Diabetes Care 2000; 23: 1278

31. Mokdad AH, Serdula MK, Dietz WH, et al. The spread of the obesity epidemic in the United States, 1991–1998. JAMA 1999; 282: 1519

32. Mokdad AH, Bowman RA, Ford ES, et al. The continuing epidemics of obesity and diabetes in the United States. JAMA 2001; 286: 1195

33. Amos AF, McCarty DJ, Zimmet P. The rising global burdens of diabetes and its complications: estimates and projections to the year 2010. Diabet Med 1997; 4 (Suppl 5): S7

34. International Diabetes Federation. Diabetes Atlas, 2nd edn. 2003

35. Obesity: preventing and managing the global epidemic. Report of a WHO Consultation. WHO Technical Report Series, No. 894. Geneva: World Health Organization, 2000

36. Evans RM, Barish GD, Wang YU. PPARs and the complex journey to obesity. Nat Med 2004; 10: 355–61

2 Insulin resistance and cardiometabolic risk

As discussed in Chapter 1, insulin resistance is defined as a clinical state in which a normal or elevated insulin level produces an impaired biological response. Specifically, the ability of insulin to enhance glucose uptake, suppress lipolysis, and decrease hepatic gluconeogenesis, in peripheral tissues, such as liver, skeletal muscle, and adipose tissue, is attenuated. The presence of insulin resistance is considered to be one of the key pathophysiological parameters associated with both obesity and type 2 diabetes, and is highly associated with traditional and non-traditional risk factors increasing cardiometabolic risk (Figure 2.1). As also observed, clinical insulin resistance can be considered as either a primary lesion of a condition, or secondary to other conditions that may attenuate insulin action, such as abnormal insulin molecules, or circulating insulin antagonists (e.g. glucocorticoids, growth hormone, anti-insulin antibodies) (Table 2.1). Insulin resistance may even be observed to be secondary to genetic syndromes such as the muscular dystrophies (Table 2.1). However, the pathophysiological parameter considered as a major contributor for increasing cardiometabolic risk represents a target-tissue (i.e. skeletal muscle) defect in insulin action and accounts for the overwhelming majority of cases of insulin resistance reported for the human condition (Table 2.1)[1].

MEASUREMENT OF INSULIN RESISTANCE AND CLINICAL ASSESSMENT

Clinically, a number of techniques have been developed to detect the presence of insulin resistance and assessments vary in complexity and precision (Figure 2.2)[2–6]. However, from a clinical perspective, the most practical way of assessing insulin resistance is the measurement of plasma insulin levels. (Insulin is produced in pancreatic β-cells and is released into the bloodstream in response to stimulation that occurs after a meal ingestion (Figures 2.3 and 2.4)[7]. As type 2 diabetes is characterized by an antecedent phase of insulin resistance that requires a compensatory increase in insulin secretion to maintain euglycemia, an elevated insulin level in the fasting state is indicative of insulin resistance.) It is suggested that this be performed in the overnight fasting condition, since in the postprandial state glucose levels are changing rapidly, and variable levels of glucose confound the simultaneous measurement of insulin. The homeostasis model assessment (HOMA)[4,5] of insulin sensitivity is a simple, inexpensive alternative to more sophisticated techniques and derives an estimate of insulin sensitivity from the mathematical modeling of fasting plasma glucose and insulin concentrations. Specifically, an estimate of insulin resistance by HOMA score is calculated with the formula: (fasting serum insulin (μU/ml) × fasting plasma glucose (mM))/22.5. Oral glucose tolerance testing (OGTT) enables the insulin secretory response to an oral glucose challenge to be calculated[6]. The frequently sampled intravenous glucose tolerance test (FSIVGTT) is a method that is less invasive and more practical than the euglycemic hyperinsulinemic clamp technique and one that can be applied to larger populations[2,3]. With this procedure, glucose is injected as a bolus, and both glucose and insulin levels are assessed frequently from an

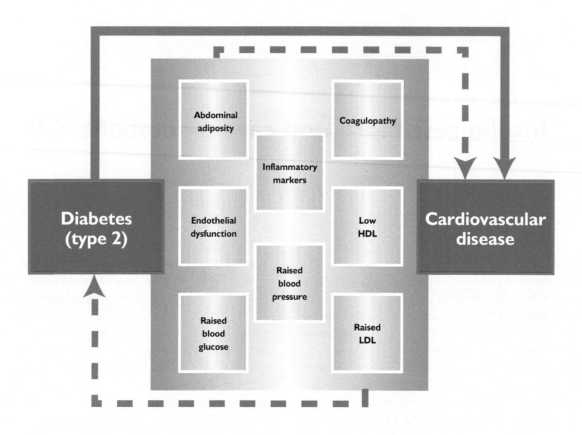

Figure 2.1   Illustration of traditional and non-traditional factors associated with cardiometabolic risk

indwelling catheter over the next several hours. The results are entered in a computer model that generates a value as an index of insulin sensitivity, termed S_I units.

The most widely accepted research gold standard is the euglycemic hyperinsulinemic clamp technique[2,3]. In this procedure, exogenous insulin is infused to maintain a constant plasma insulin level above fasting, whereas glucose is infused at varying rates to keep glucose within a fixed range. The amount of glucose that is infused over time (*M* value) is an index of insulin action on glucose metabolism. As described, the more glucose that has to be infused per unit time to maintain the fixed blood glucose level, the more sensitive the patient is to insulin. With this procedure, the insulin-resistant patient requires much less infused glucose to maintain the basal level of glucose. Studies that have used any or all of these techniques have

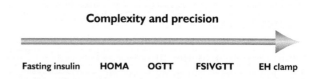

Figure 2.2   Techniques used to assess insulin resistance. HOMA, homeostasis model assessment; OGTT, oral glucose tolerance test; FSIVGTT, frequently sampled intravenous glucose tolerance test; EH clamp, euglycemic hyperinsulinemic clamp

demonstrated that there is a wide range of insulin sensitivity in normal individuals, and that these levels may overlap with values obtained in subjects with type 2

Table 2.1 Human diseases and conditions characterized by insulin resistance. From reference 1, with permission

Insulin resistance may be primary	Insulin resistance may be secondary	Insulin resistance associated with genetic syndromes
Type 2 diabetes mellitus	Obesity	Progeroid syndromes (e.g. Werner's syndrome)
Insulin resistance syndrome (syndrome X)	Type I diabetes mellitus	Cytogenetic disorders (Down's, Turner's, and Klinefelter's)
Gestational diabetes mellitus	Type B severe insulin resistance	Ataxia telangiectasia
Type A severe insulin resistance	Hyperlipidemias	Muscular dystrophies
Lipoatrophic diabetes	Pregnancy	Friedreich's ataxia
Leprechaunism	Acute illness and stress	Alstrom syndrome
Rabson–Mendenhall syndrome	Cushing's disease and syndrome	Laurence–Moon–Biedl syndrome
Hypertension	Pheochromocytoma	Pseudo-Refsum's syndrome
Atherosclerotic cardiovascular disease	Acromegaly	Other rare hereditary neuromuscular disorders
	Hyperthyroidism	
	Liver cirrhosis	
	Renal failure	

diabetes. Furthermore, even at similar levels of body mass index (BMI), there appear to be ethnic differences in the degree of insulin sensitivity (Figure 2.5)[8]. Therefore, it is very difficult to distinguish between non-diabetic and diabetic individuals on the basis of insulin resistance.

RELATIONSHIP OF INSULIN RESISTANCE TO CLINICAL RISK FACTORS AND CARDIOVASCULAR DISEASE

The relationship of insulin resistance to the factors that increase cardiometabolic risk is not in question (Figure 2.6)[9]. The cardiometabolic risk syndrome represents a clustering of risk factors associated with insulin resistance and obesity which contributes significantly to the development of cardiovascular disease. Cause and effect are difficult to establish, and significant interaction exists between multiple risk factors.

Obesity

Insulin resistance is frequently observed in obese subjects and has been established as an independent risk factor for the development of both type 2 diabetes and coronary artery disease[10–13]. Although it is established that hyperinsulinemia, insulin resistance, and other obesity-related metabolic abnormalities are significantly associated with overall accumulation of fat in the body, there is now substantial evidence that the specific distribution of fat is important as outlined in Chapter 3. Excessive accumulation of fat in the upper body's so-called truncal region, or central obesity, is a better predictor of morbidity than excess fat in the lower body, the so-called lower body segment obesity[10,12,13].

Glucose metabolism

Abnormalities in glucose tolerance are commonly noted in individuals with central obesity. As outlined in Chapter 1, it is now well accepted that the presence of insulin resistance in an individual will need to be compensated for by hyperinsulinemia in order to maintain normal glucose tolerance. In those individuals who develop diabetes, a progressive loss of the insulin secretory capacity fails to compensate for the insulin resistance and results in a progressive hyperglycemia (see Chapter 1). Thus, an individual with obesity and insulin resistance, depending on the stage of compensation for the insulin resistance, may have euglycemia, impaired fasting glucose, impaired glucose tolerance, or overt hyperglycemia confirming the diagnosis of type 2 diabetes.

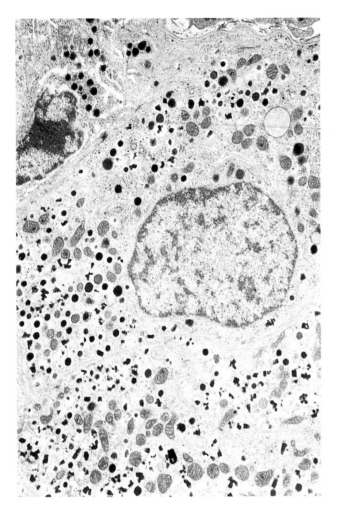

Figure 2.3 Electron micrograph of an islet of Langerhans from a normal pancreas showing mainly insulin storage granules in a pancreatic β-cell. A larger α (glucagon) cell is also seen. The normal adult pancreas contains around one million islets comprising mainly β-cells (producing insulin), α-cells (glucagon), D cells (somatostatin), and PP (pancreatic polypeptide) cells. From reference 7, with permission

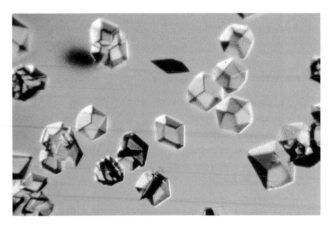

Figure 2.4 Insulin crystals. Insulin is stored in β-cells as hexamers complexed with zinc. Insulin–zinc hexamers readily form crystals which are stored in the pancreatic granules. In the blood, insulin is not seen in aggregated forms such as dimers or hexamers, but as monomers which are formed when insulin granules are liberated. From reference 7 with permission

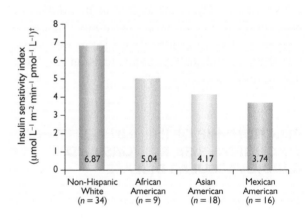

Figure 2.5 Insulin sensitivity among different ethic groups (age 23–26 years, BMI 23–26.5 kg/m^2). $^*p = 0.002$ vs. Caucasians; †data are geometric means. From reference 8 with permission

Lipid abnormalities

Unfavorable changes in lipoproteins, in part, may help explain the increased risk for cardiovascular disease observed with insulin-resistant states[14–18]. One of the major quantitative changes observed in insulin-resistant states is an elevation in triglyceride-rich lipoproteins. This is often accompanied by a decreased HDL cholesterol level[16]. Thus, the characteristic lipid abnormalities (by association with insulin resistance) may be observed long before the diagnosis of type 2 diabetes. Although LDL cholesterol levels may be comparable to those seen in the general population, LDL compositional differences may make these particles more atherogenic. Specifically, insulin-resistant states are significantly associated with both quantitative changes (e.g. increased triglycerides, high apolipoprotein (apo)B, low apoA1 levels) in the lipoproteins and also qualitative changes (e.g. low LDL cholesterol/apoB

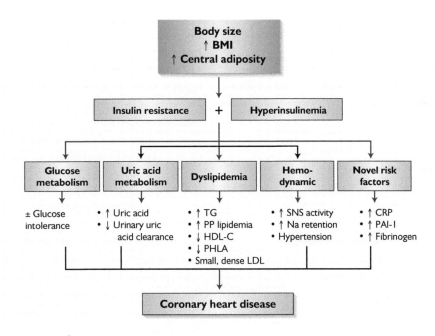

Figure 2.6 Current perspectives and relationship of insulin resistance to cardiovascular risk factors and disease. TG, triglyceride; PP, postprandial; PHLA, postheparin lipolytic activity; SNS, sympathetic nervous system; CRP, C-reactive protein; PAI-1, plasminogen-activator inhibitor-1. From reference 9 with permission

and low HDL cholesterol/low apoA1)[16,19]. Insulin resistance has also been associated with this preponderance of small dense LDL particles, and it is the small dense LDL particle that has been suggested to be the more atherogenic LDL[14,15].

Hypertension

Hemodynamic abnormalities such as hypertension are key contributors to increasing cardiovascular risk. The etiology of hypertension in the metabolic syndrome is complex and multifactorial. Evidence has suggested that obesity, insulin resistance, and dyslipidemia all contribute to the development of hypertension. Obesity, in particular, may play the largest role in creating the conditions that lead to hypertension as part of the cardiometabolic risk syndrome[20].

Non-traditional risk factors

Recently there has been substantial evidence showing a relationship between non-traditional risk factors and insulin resistance. These factors include inflammatory markers, such as C-reactive protein, and markers

assessing a hypercoagulable state, such as the plasminogen-activator inhibitors, e.g. PAI-1. These non-traditional risk factors are covered in detail in other chapters of this Atlas.

Endothelial dysfunction

The vascular endothelium has received considerable research attention based on its primary role in modulating the underlying blood vessel tone by producing a number of factors. These factors include vasoconstrictors, vasodilators, in addition to agents involved in inflammatory and fibrinolytic pathways (Table 2.2). Agents that preferentially dilate the vascular wall include nitric oxide (NO), prostacyclin, bradykinin, and endothelium-derived hyperpolarization factor. Agents that have been found to constrict blood vessel tone include endothelin, superoxide anion, endothelium-derived constricting factor, locally produced angiotensin II, and thromboxane. These agents have been described not only to control and regulate arterial tone, but also to affect other parameters that contribute to the development of atherosclerosis[21–23]. From the above discussion, therefore, it can be appreciated that the endothelium has great potential to participate in cell proliferation contributing to the development and progression of atherosclerosis.

It is now well described that endothelial dysfunction may be secondary to insulin resistance and hyperinsulinemia, in addition to other components of the cardiometabolic syndrome (Figure 2.7)[21–23]. Hyperlipidemia, hyperglycemia, hypertension, smoking, and homocysteine have all been reported to damage the endothelium. (Studies that have treated these particular components have also shown favorable effects on endothelial dysfunction). Endothelial dysfunction leads to an imbalance in the endothelial production of favorable versus unfavorable factors. Factors such as platelet adhesion, aggregation, and thrombogenicity of the blood have been postulated to play a role. Therefore, secondary to endothelial dysfunction, circulating platelets may aggregate in particular areas, releasing cytokines and growth factors, and may initiate the inflammatory reaction. After the initial inflammatory reaction, LDL cholesterol is postulated to be more actively taken up into the vessel wall and may result in the formation of a fatty streak. Ultimately, vascular smooth muscle cells participate in the process by migrating into the intima, proliferating, and increasing their production of extracellular matrix proteins. The summation of these processes results in organized atherosclerotic plaque formation[21–23]. Studies that have assessed endothelial function have suggested that endothelial function is decreased in individuals with impaired glucose tolerance, diabetes or relatives of these individuals[24] (Figure 2.8).

Table 2.2 Factors released by endothelium. Compiled from references 21–23

Vasoactive substances
- Vasodilators
  - Nitric oxide/EDRF
  - EDHF
  - Prostacyclin (PGI$_2$)
  - Bradykinin
  - Acetylcholine, serotonin, histamine, substance P, etc.

- Vasoconstrictors
  - Endothelin
  - Angiotensin II
  - Thromboxane A$_2$, acetylcholine, arachidonic acid, prostaglandin H$_2$, etc.

Growth mediators/modulators
- Growth promoters
- Growth inhibitors

Inflammatory mediators/ modulators
- TNF-α
- IL-6
- CRP

Hemostasis and thrombosis
- PAI-1

Redox state
- ROS

EDRF, endothelium-derived relaxing factor; EDHF, endothelium-derived hyperpolarizing factor; TNF-α, tumor necrosis factor α; IL-6, interleukin-6; CRP, C-reactive protein; PAI-1, plasminogen-activator inhibitor-1; ROS, reactive oxygen species

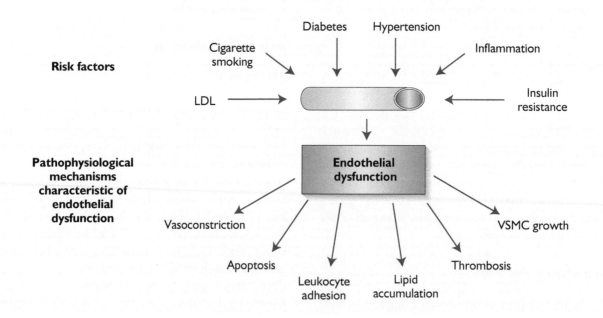

Figure 2.7 Traditional and non-traditional risk factors contributing to endothelial dysfunction. VSMC, vascular smooth muscle cell

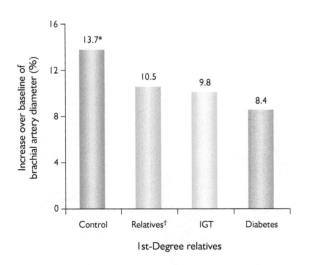

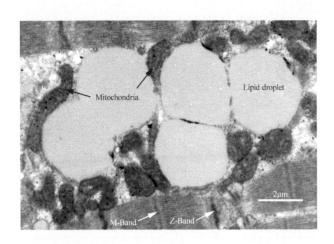

Defining the cellular lesion

Understanding the cellular mechanism(s) that contribute to insulin resistance is important in identifying its genetic basis and would allow both the development of effective therapies and optimal use of current therapies. As outlined in Chapter 4, we know that obesity and insulin resistance are associated with increases in intramyocellular lipids (Figure 2.9). From

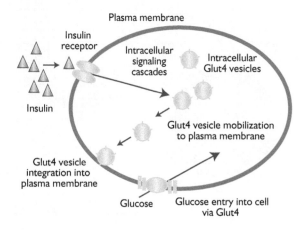

Figure 2.8 Impaired endothelium-dependent vasodilatation in individuals at risk for type 2 diabetes. IGT, impaired glucose tolerance; $*p < 0.01$, control vs. relatives, IGT, diabetes; [†]one or both parents. From reference 24, with permission

Figure 2.10 Insulin stimulated glucose uptake in muscle and fat cells. Illustration shows mobilization of Glut4 (glucose transporter 4) to the cell surface. After insulin binding to the receptor and generation of the second messengers for insulin action, glucose transport into the cell is activated. This effect of insulin is brought about by the translocation of a large pool of glucose transporters from an intracellular pool to the plasma membrane. The glucose transport proteins have distinct specificities, kinetic properties, and tissue distribution that define their clinical role. Two major glut proteins (Glut1 and 4) have been identified in skeletal muscle; Glut1 may be involved primarily in basal glucose uptake, whereas the major insulin-responsive glucose transporter isoform is termed Glut4 and is predominantly expressed in insulin target tissues such as skeletal and cardiac muscle and adipose tissue. In normal muscle cells, Glut4 is recycled between the plasma membrane and intracellular storage pools; thus, it differs from other transporters in that 90% of it is sequestered intracellularly in the absence of insulin. With insulin stimulation, the equilibrium of this recycling process is altered to favor translocation (regulated movement) of Glut4 from intracellular stores to the plasma membrane and transverse tubules in the muscle, resulting in a rise in the maximal velocity of glucose transport into the cell. Courtesy of Dr Derek Leroith, MD

Figure 2.9 Obesity and insulin resistance are associated with increases in intramyocellular lipid accumulation. This figure represents an electron micrograph (EM) of human skeletal muscle. As outlined, the EM demonstrates muscle fibers, mitochondria and lipid droplets within the muscle cell. The mechanism of the deposition of lipids in muscle is outlined in Chapter 4. Courtesy of Enette Larson-Meyer with special thanks to Tressa M Penrod for photo touching

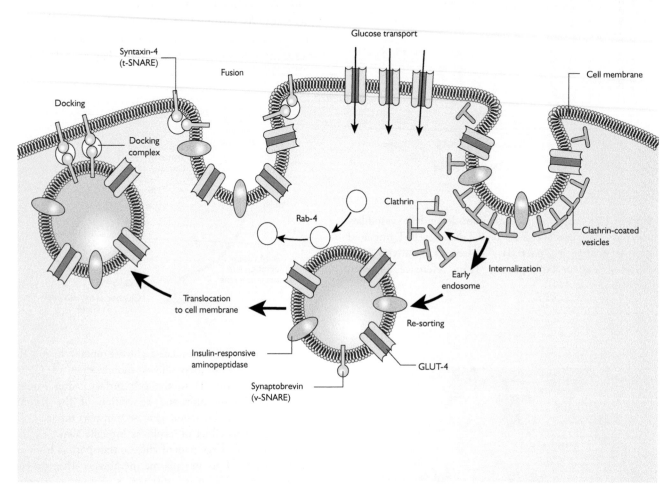

Figure 2.11 Mechanisms involved in the translocation of GLUT-4 glucose transporters in muscle cells and adipocytes. In the absence of insulin, about 90% of GLUT-4 is sequestered intracellularly in distinct vesicles that also contain proteins such as insulin-responsive aminopeptidase, synaptobrevin (also known as vesicle-associated membrane protein-2, or v-SNARE), and the small guanosine triphosphate-binding protein Rab-4. In response to insulin, exercise, or contraction, vesicles containing GLUT-4 move to the plasma membrane, where they dock, forming complexes involving syntaxin-4 (also known as target synaptosome-associated protein receptor, or t-SNARE) and synaptobrevin. The vesicles fuse with the plasma membrane, increasing the number of GLUT-4 molecules in the membrane and thus the rate of glucose transport into cells. Rab-4 leaves the vesicle and moves into the cytosol in response to insulin stimulation. On removal of insulin stimulation, GLUT-4 is internalized by the budding of clathrin-coated vesicles from the plasma membrane. GLUT-4 enters early endosomes, from which it is re-sorted to intracellular GLUT-4-containing vesicles. From reference 31, with permission

a clinical perspective, the aspect of insulin resistance that has been most studied is defective insulin-mediated glucose uptake and utilization in response to insulin stimulation in insulin-sensitive tissues[25–27]. In patients, this defect is manifested by a reduction in glycogen synthesis in muscle and liver[28].

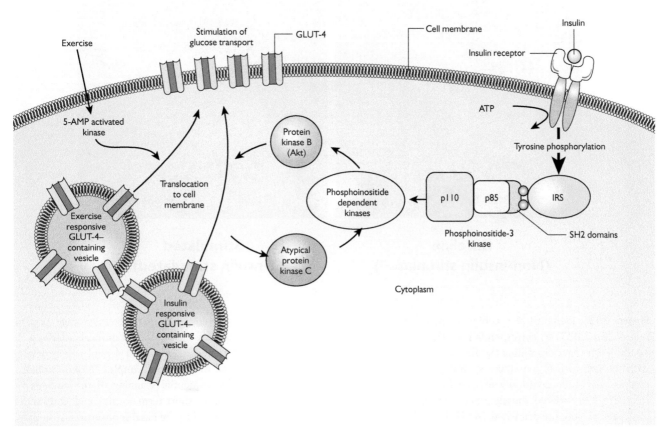

Figure 2.12 Insulin signaling pathways that regulate glucose metabolism in muscle cells and adipocytes. GLUT-4 is stored in intracellular vesicles. Insulin binds to its receptor in the plasma membrane, resulting in phosphorylation of the receptor and insulin-receptor substrates such as the IRS molecules. These substrates form complexes with docking proteins such as phosphoinositide-3 kinase at its 85-kDa subunit (p85) by means of SH2 (Scr homology region 2) domains. Then p85 is constitutively bound to the catalytic subunit (p110). Activation of phosphoinositide-3 kinase is a major pathway in the mediation of insulin-stimulated glucose transport and metabolism. It activates phosphoinositide-dependant kinases that participate in the activation of protein kinase B (also known as Akt) and atypical forms of protein kinase C (PKC). Exercise stimulates glucose transport by pathways that are independent of phosphoinositide-3 kinase and that may involve 5'-AMP-activated kinase. From reference 31, with permission

Insulin action in insulin-sensitive peripheral tissues (e.g. fat or muscle) begins with specific binding to high-affinity receptors on the plasma membrane of the target tissue. This binding activates the receptor and generates second messengers which are responsible for initiating many cellular processes that define the biological action of insulin, including the uptake of glucose into the cell[29,30] (Figures 2.10–2.13). The cellular abnormality accounting for clinical insulin resistance theoretically could involve any one of the multiple steps of the insulin-signaling cascade, as alterations in insulin production, insulin binding, or intracellular signaling all have the potential to induce an insulin-resistant state. The insulin resistance most commonly observed clinically is referred to as a postreceptor defect because insulin signaling and/or effective glucose transport after insulin binding (i.e. intracellular events) is attenuated.

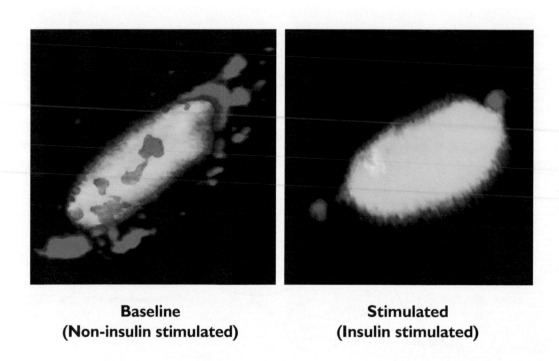

**Baseline
(Non-insulin stimulated)**

**Stimulated
(Insulin stimulated)**

Figure 2.13 Demonstrates confocal microscopic imaging protocol to reproducibly measure a transient storage pool of perinuclear GLUT-4, corresponding to the trans-Golgi network in human skeletal muscle biopsies. Confocal images were assembled by first examining the flat plane, and focusing on regions where the immunoreactive GLUT-4 pool was associated with the perinuclear zone (corresponding to the trans-Golgi network) of the skeletal muscle fiber sample. These perinuclear regions were then confocally imaged for GLUT-4 in the depth plane followed by sequential scanning of the nucleus for reference. On isolated muscle fibers. this pool has been shown to be depleted upon short-term insulin and contraction stimulation. Note the decreased GLUT 4 signal (red) in the insulin stimulated as compared to the basal (non-insulin stimulated state) muscle biopsy. Red, perinuclear GLUT 4; green, skeletal muscle nucleus. Courtesy of Dr Tom Jetton

REFERENCES

1. Hunter SJ, Garvey WT. Insulin action and insulin resistance: diseases involving defects in insulin receptors, signal transduction, and the glucose transport effector system. Am J Med 1998; 105: 331–45

2. Ferrannini E, Mari A. How to measure insulin sensitivity. J Hypertens 1998; 16: 895–906

3. Del Prato S. Measurement of insulin resistance in vivo. Drugs 1999; 58 (Suppl 1): 3–6

4. Bonora E, Targher G, Alberiche M, et al. Homeostasis model assessment closely mirrors the glucose clamp technique in the assessment of insulin sensitivity. Diabetes Care 2000; 23: 57–63

5. Matthews DR, Hosker JP, Rudenski AS, et al. Homeostasis model assessment: insulin resistance and β-cell function from fasting plasma glucose and insulin concentrations in man. Diabetologia 1985; 28: 412–19

6. Yeni-Komshian H, Carantoni M, Abbasi F, Reaven GM. Relationship between several surrogate estimates of insulin resistance and quantification of insulin-mediated glucose disposal in 490 healthy nondiabetic volunteers. Diabetes Care 2000; 23: 171–5

7. Scobie IN. An Atlas of Diabetes Mellitus, 2nd edn. London: Parthenon Publishing, 2002

8. Chiu KC, Cohan P, Lee NP, Chuang LM. Insulin sensitivity differs among ethnic groups with a compensatory response in beta-cell function. Diabetes Care 2000; 23: 1353–8

9. Reaven G. Syndrome X: 10 years after. Drugs 1999; 58 (Suppl 1):19–20

10. Abate N. Insulin resistance and obesity: the role of fat distribution pattern. Diabetes Care 1996; 19: 292–4

11. Howard G, O'Leary DH, Zaccaro D, et al. Insulin sensitivity and atherosclerosis: The Insulin Resistance Atherosclerosis Study (IRAS) Investigators. Circulation 1996; 93: 1809–17

12. Kaplan NM. The deadly quartet. Upper-body obesity, glucose intolerance, hypertriglyceridemia, and hypertension. Arch Intern Med 1989; 149: 1514–20

13. Yamashita S, Nakamura T, Shimomura I, et al. Insulin resistance and body fat distribution. Diabetes Care 1996; 19: 287–91

14. Grundy SM. Small LDL, atherogenic dyslipidemia, and the metabolic syndrome. Circulation 1997; 95: 1–4

15. Fagan TC, Deedwania PC. The cardiovascular dysmetabolic syndrome. Am J Med 1998; 105: 77–82S

16. Grundy SM. Hypertriglyceridemia, insulin resistance, and the metabolic syndrome. Am J Cardiol 1999; 83: 25F–9F

17. Lamarche B, Lemieux I, Despres JP. The small, dense LDL phenotype and the risk of coronary heart disease: epidemiology, pathophysiology, and therapeutic aspects. Diabetes Metab 1999; 25: 199–211

18. Sheu WH, Jeng CY, Young MS, et al. Coronary artery disease risk predicted by insulin resistance, plasma lipids, and hypertension in people without diabetes. Am J Med Sci 2000; 319: 84–8

19. MacLean PS, Vadlamudi S, MacDonald KG, et al. Impact of insulin resistance on lipoprotein subpopulation distribution in lean and morbidly obese nondiabetic women. Metabolism 2000; 49: 285–92

20. Hall JE, Brands MW, Henegar JR. Mechanisms of hypertension and kidney disease in obesity. Ann NY Acad Sci 1999; 107: 91–107

21. Hsueh WA, Quinones MJ, Creager MA. Endothelium in insulin resistance and diabetes. Diabetes Rev 1997; 5: 343–52

22. Hsueh WA, Law RE. Cardiovascular risk continuum: implications of insulin resistance and diabetes. Am J Med 1998; 105: 4S–14S

23. Quyyumi AA. Endothelial function in health and disease: new insights into the genesis of cardiovascular disease. Am J Med 1998; 105: 32S–9S

24. Caballero AE, et al. Microvascular and macrovascular reactivity is reduced in subjects at risk for type 2 diabetes. Diabetes. 1999; 48: 1856–62

25. Reaven GM. Bantin lecture 1988: role of insulin resistance in human disease. Diabetes 1988; 37: 1595–607

26. Shulman GI. Cellular mechanisms of insulin resistance in humans. Am J Cardiol 1999; 84: 3–10J

27. Cline GW, Petersen KF, Krssak M, et al. Impaired glucose transport as a cause of decreased insulin-stimulated muscle glycogen synthesis in type II diabetes. N Engl J Med 1999; 341: 240–6

28. Beck-Nielsen H. Mechanisms of insulin resistance in non-oxidative glucose metabolism: the role of glycogen synthase. J Basic Clin Physiol Pharmacol 1998; 9: 255–79

29. White MF, Kahn CR. The insulin signaling system. J Biol Chem 1994; 269: 1–4

30. Cheatham B, Kahn CR. Insulin action and the insulin signaling network. Endocr Rev 1995; 16: 117–42

31. Shepherd PR, Kahn BB. Glucose transporters and insulin action: implications for insulin resistance and diabetes mellitus. N Engl J Med 1999; 341: 248–57

3 Role of obesity and body fat distribution in cardiometabolic risk

Obesity can be simply defined as an excessive amount of body fat which increases the risk of medical illness and premature death. For clinical purposes, assessments that are routinely used to define obesity include body weight and body mass index (BMI)[1]. The BMI assessment represents the relationship between weight and height, and is derived by calculating either the weight (in kg) divided by the height (in meters squared), or the weight (in pounds) multiplied by 704 divided by the height in inches squared[1]. Using the BMI as the main criteria, classification of obesity into risk categories have been proposed (Table 3.1). The BMI classification is based on data that has been collected from large epidemiological studies that evaluated body weight and mortality[2–4]. This classification provides clinicians with a mechanism for identifying patients at high risk for complications associated with obesity. It has been well established that those individuals considered obese, i.e. BMI ≥ 30, are at much higher risk for cardiovascular mortality than those considered overweight, i.e. BMI between 25 and 29.9[1] (Figure 3.1).

The prevalence of obesity has reached epidemic proportions around the world and the rate continues to increase. According to the World Health Organization (WHO), it has been estimated that over 1 billion adults worldwide are overweight and at least 300 million are considered obese[5]. Many factors contribute to this rise, but among the major factors are sedentary lifestyles, consumption of high-fat caloric-dense diets, and increased urbanization. In the US alone, data from the National Health and Nutrition Examination Surveys obtained since 1960 have suggested that over

Table 3.1 BMI-associated disease risk. Reproduced from reference 1, with permission

	Obesity class	BMI (kg/m^2)	Risk
Underweight		< 18.5	Increased
Normal		18.5–24.9	Normal
Overweight		25.0–29.9	Increased
Obesity	I	30.0–34.9	High
	II	35.0–39.9	Very high
Extreme obesity	III	≥ 40	Extremely high

Additional risks: (1) waist circumference > 40 inches in men and > 35 inches in women; (2) weight gain of ≥ 5 kg since age 18–20 years; (3) poor aerobic fitness; and (4) Southeast Asian descent

64% of the US adult population is classified as either overweight or obese (BMI > 25)[5]. Whereas the prevalence of overweight adults has increased slightly, from approximately 30.5% to 34.0%, the prevalence of obesity (BMI ≥ 30) has more than doubled from approximately 13% in 1960 to over 30% in the year 2000[5]. Furthermore, the prevalence of individuals with extreme obesity as defined by a BMI ≥ 40 has increased over 6-fold in the same 40-year period (0.8% vs. 4.7%)[5]. Most of the increase in body weight has occurred since 1980 and, unfortunately, this trend is not expected to change (Figure 3.2[6]). Thus, we will have to address the economic, medical, and psychosocial consequences of this epidemic for years to come.

Obviously, the major concern associated with the obesity epidemic centers around the associated

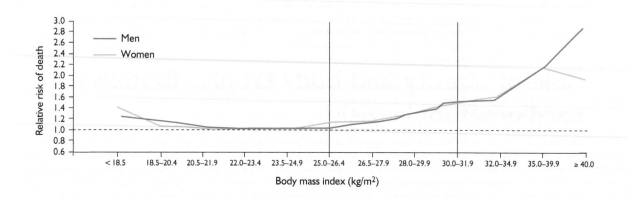

Figure 3.1 Relationship between body mass index (BMI) and cardiovascular mortality in 302 233 adult men and women who had never smoked and had no pre-existing illness. Vertical lines indicate cut-off values for over-weight and obese of BMI 25.0–29.9 kg/m² and obese BMI ≥ 30 kg/m², respectively. From reference 3, with permission

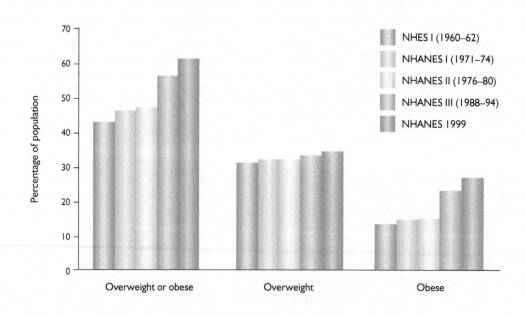

Figure 3.2 Age adjusted prevalence of overweight (BMI 25–29 kg/m²) and obesity (BMI ≥ 30 kg/m²) in adults aged 20–74 years in the US since 1960. Data were obtained from the four National Health and Nutrition Examination surveys conducted between 1960 and 2000. As shown, the prevalence of overweight individuals has increased slightly, but the prevalence of obesity has more than doubled. From reference 1, with permission. Data from reference 6 and National Center for Health Statistics, Centers for Disease Control and Prevention website www.cdc.gov/nchs/products/pubs/pubd/hestats/obese/obse99.htm

complications which seem to affect every major organ system (Table 3.2). Specifically, obesity increases an individual's risk for cancer, gastrointestinal diseases, arthritis, and adversely affects psychological well-being. However, the major concern, as described in detail in this Atlas, is the markedly increased risk to develop diabetes and cardiovascular disease in those individuals who are obese. Specifically, obesity is significantly associated with both the traditional risk factors, i.e. hypertension, dyslipidemia, diabetes, and the non-traditional risk factors, i.e. fibrinogen and inflammatory markers, of cardiovascular disease. In addition,

as the presence of insulin resistance is considered as the hallmark for the presence of the cardiometabolic risk syndrome, it is clear that obesity and insulin resistance are integrally related (Figure 3.3).

BODY FAT DISTRIBUTION

The traditional view of adipose tissue is simply a reservoir for desposition of excess calories only has not been valid for years. It is very true that adipocytes serve as a major tissue for energy storage and there is

Table 3.2 Medical complications associated with obesity. From reference 1, with permission

Gastrointestinal	Gallstones, pancreatitis, abdominal hernia, NAFLD* (steatosis, steatohepatitis, and cirrhosis), and possibly GERD†
Endocrine/metabolic	Metabolic syndrome, insulin resistance, impaired glucose tolerance, type 2 diabetes mellitus, dyslipidemia, polycystic ovary syndrome
Cardiovascular	Hypertension, coronary heart disease, congestive heart failure, dysrhythmias, pulmonary hypertension, ischemic stroke, venous stasis, deep vein thrombosis, pulmonary embolus
Respiratory	Abnormal pulmonary function, obstructive sleep apnea, obesity hypoventilation syndrome
Musculoskeletal	Osteoarthritis, gout, low back pain
Gyneocologic	Abnormal menses, infertility
Genitourinary	Urinary stress incontinence
Ophthalmologic	Cataracts
Neurologic	Idiopathic intracranial hypertension (pseudotumor cerebri)
Cancer	Esophagus, colon, gallbladder, prostate, breast, uterus, cervix, kidney
Postoperative events	Atelectasis, pneumonia, deep vein thrombosis, pulmonary embolus

*Non-alcoholic fatty liver disease; †gastroesophageal reflux disease

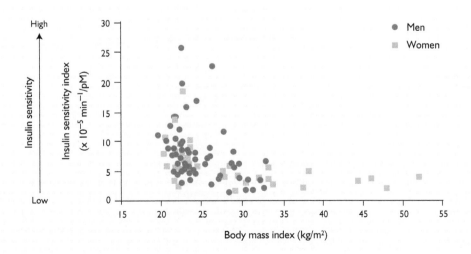

Figure 3.3 Relationship of insulin sensitivity to body mass index. With increasing obesity as assessed by the increase in BMI, obese individuals are characterized as insulin resistant, whereas lean individuals with BMI < 25 may be markedly insulin sensitive. From reference 7, with permission

a growing science demonstrating that size, differentiation, and secretions from the adipocyte are all important functions[8–10] (Figure 3.4).

Individuals who are obese and have a high concentration of visceral adipose tissue tend to have dyslipidemia in the form of elevated levels of triglycerides and decreased levels of high-density lipoprotein cholesterol (HDL-C), which place them at higher risk for cardiovascular disease. As obesity is a major factor to increase metabolic risk, the relevancy of managing obesity to prevent and/or ameliorate chronic diseases such as cardiovascular disease and type 2 diabetes is undeniable[11].

The body weight and BMI have served an important purpose in stratifying individuals at high risk. However, the assessment of the specific distribution of the body fat may be considered an even more important assessment. In past studies, body fat distribution has been generally assessed by anthropometric measurements consisting of waist circumference, the waist-to-hip ratio (WHR), or skin fold thicknesses (Figure 3.5). When using skin fold measures, the most commonly utilized has been the subscapular-to-triceps ratio, or a sum of central-to-peripheral skinfolds[12]. Regardless of which is utilized, these measures are used to classify the subject as having either upper body, i.e. 'central' or abdominal obesity, or lower body obesity. In lay terms, these body types have been referred to as the 'apple-' or 'pear-shape' phenotypes (Figure 3.6). Abdominal adiposity, in addition to being significantly associated with the metabolic abnormalities that constitute the cardiometabolic syndrome, is

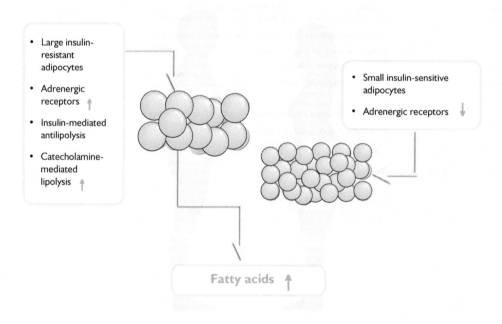

Figure 3.4 There is strong evidence suggesting adipose tissue has a central role in contributing to insulin resistance. New evidence suggests that insulin resistance is partly the result of the inability of the adipose organ to expand to accommodate excess calories. Increased fat cell size may represent the failure of the adipose tissue mass to expand, i.e. proliferate and differentiate, resulting in a reduced ability to accommodate an increased energy influx. When combined with reduced fat oxidation in adipose tissue, these pathophysiologic changes will contribute to a decrease in fat storage in adipocytes and an increase peripheral deposition of lipids in tissues, i.e. increased 'ectopic fat'. Individuals who have a low capacity for proliferation and/or differentiation of precursors into mature fat-storing adipocytes are susceptible to hypertrophy of the existing adipocytes under conditions of energy excess. Thus, adipocyte hypertrophy (i.e. large fat cells) is indicative of a failure to proliferate and/or differentiate; a failure to accommodate an increased energy flux resulting in ectopic (intracellular) storage in sites such as muscle, liver and pancreas; and correlates better with insulin resistance than with any other measure of adiposity. Courtesy of Center for Obesity Research and Education

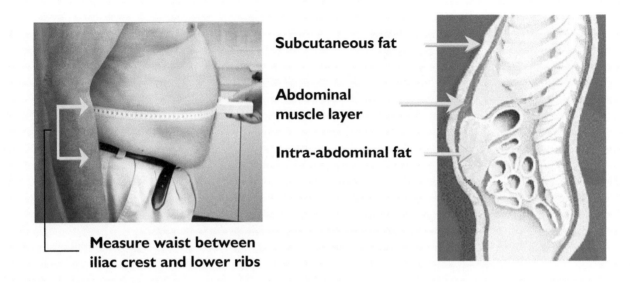

Figure 3.5 Visceral adiposity: the critical adipose depot. Epidemiologic and metabolic studies conducted over the past 15 years have noted that complications frequently found in obese patients appear to be associated with the location of excess fat rather than to excess weight per se, specifically abdominally distributed obesity. The patient with abdominal obesity, or excess visceral adipose tissue, has a high cardiometabolic risk. A simple and practical screening tool such as a measurement of the waist circumference can be used to assess risk by monitoring the accumulation or loss of visceral fat between office visits. Courtesy of Center for Obesity Research and Education

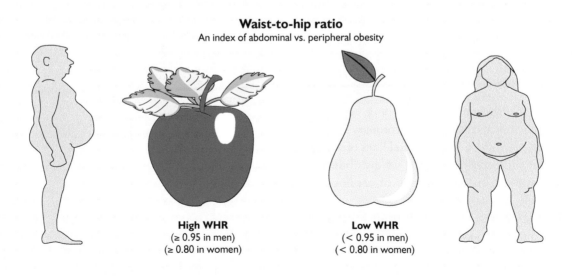

Figure 3.6 Schematic demonstrating use of anthropometric measures such as waist-to-hip ratio (WHR) in classifying central or upper-body (abdominal) obesity ('apple-shaped') versus lower-body peripheral obesity ('pear-shaped')

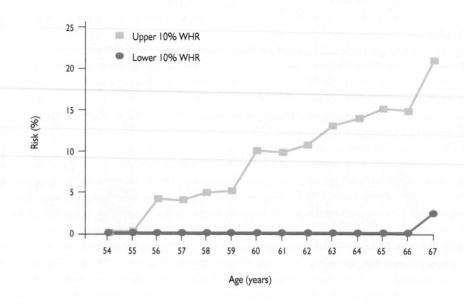

Figure 3.7   Risk of diabetes mellitus during 13 years in relation to WHR at baseline. Comparison between risk in upper and lower 10% of WHR distribution. From reference 16, with permission

also considered to be a significant risk factor for coronary heart disease in both men and women[14–16]. There is disagreement, however, between some investigators, whether this relationship holds after adjusting for total adiposity, as measured by BMI. It has been shown, however, that use of a very easily measured clinical tool such as waist circumference or WHR appears to be highly associated with development of type 2 diabetes (Figure 3.7 and Table 3.3). As it relates to cardiovascular mortality, there appears to be significant evidence that although obesity *per se* is well recognized to be a major risk factor for coronary heart disease in both men and women, several lines of evidence suggest that measures of regional fat distribution are independently associated with risk of cardiovascular disease (Table 3.3 and Figure 3.8).

In the recent past, more sophisticated techniques, such as computed tomography (CT) or magnetic resonance imaging (MRI) scans, have been utilized to assess central obesity. The advantage of these techniques is apparent in that specific and precise quantification of abdominal fat depots can be readily assessed (Figure 3.9)[12,13]. Specifically, with use of these techniques, the amount of visceral or intra-abdominal fat can be compared with the amount of

Table 3.3   The use of waist sizes in both men and women were highly associated with disease risk. Specifically, a waist circumference of 40 inches, as opposed to 37 inches, in men was associated with a 4-fold greater risk for development of type 2 diabetes and a 3–4-fold greater risk for any cardiovascular event. Similar findings were noted for women comparing waist circumference of 34 inches versus 31 inches. Data from reference 17, with permission

Men: waist size > 40 vs. < 37 inches

Women: waist size > 34 vs. < 31 inches

    4-fold greater risk for type 2 diabetes

    3- to 4-fold greater risk for major cardiovascular event

subcutaneous fat at the same level or 'cut' of the scan[12]. As such, it is now possible to appreciate the differences in fat depots in the abdominal area (Figure 3.10). Using these techniques, the relationship between fat distribution, e.g. visceral fat depots, and peripheral muscle insulin resistance has been shown to be highly correlated in both men and women (Figures 3.11–3.13)[19–21]. The pathophysiologic basis as to why central obesity, and particularly visceral fat,

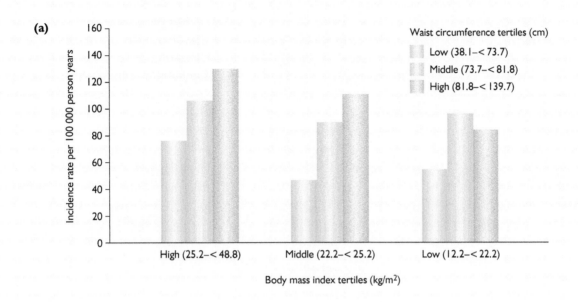

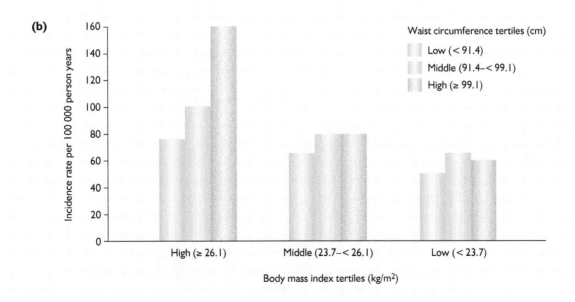

Figure 3.8 Age-adjusted incidence rates for coronary heart disease according to body mass index and waist circumference tertiles for women (a) and men (b), and according to body mass index and waist-to-hip ratio tertiles for women (c) and men (d). Adapted from references 14 and 15, with permission

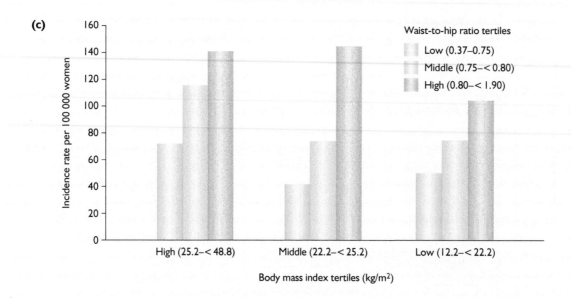

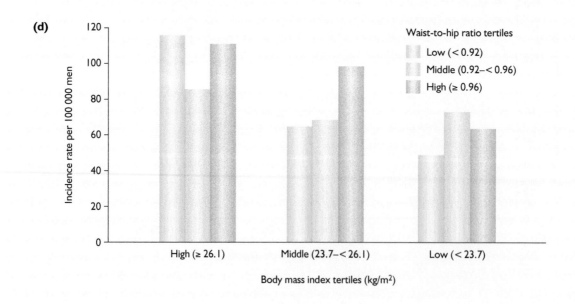

Figure 3.8 *Continued*

a

Distribution of abdominal fat deposits

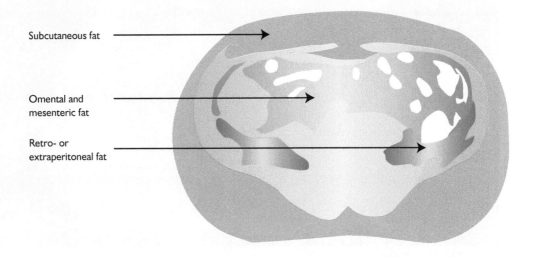

Subcutaneous fat

Omental and
mesenteric fat

Retro- or
extraperitoneal fat

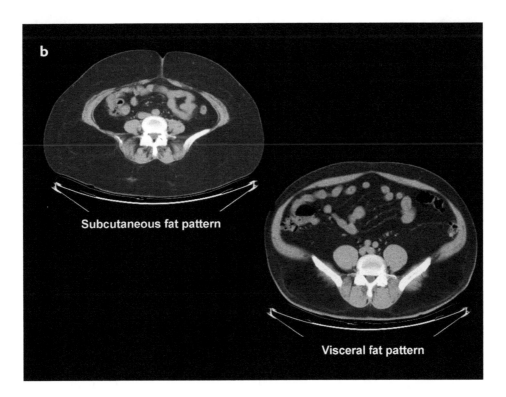

Figure 3.9 (a) Schematic demonstrating abdominal fat depots that can be measured using NMR or CT scans. (b) Scan showing subcutaneous fat and visceral fat patterning. Courtesy of Dr Steven Smith, from reference 13, with permission

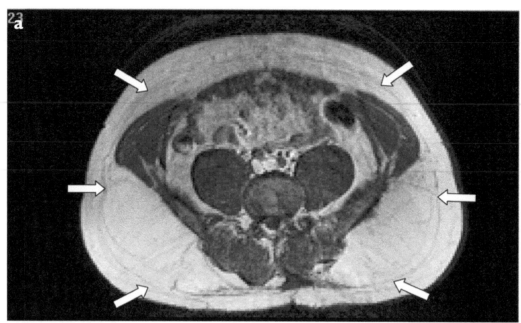

BW = 107 kg; BMI = 32.6 kg/m^2
VF = 76 cm^2; SF = 391 cm^2; DSF = 201 cm^2; SSF = 190 cm^2

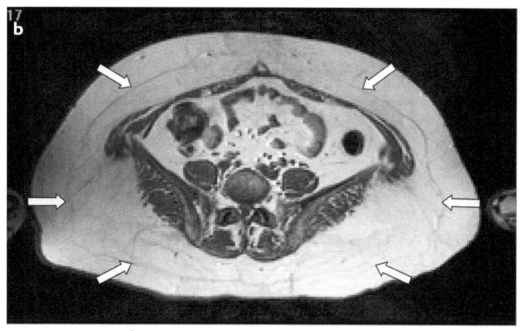

BW = 79 kg; BMI = 32.9 kg/m^2
VF = 114 cm^2; SF = 530 cm^2; DSF = 262 cm^2; SSF = 268 cm^2

Figure 3.10 Magnetic resonance imaging (MRI) of distribution of abdominal fat demonstrating transverse cross-sectional magnetic resonance image at the L4–6 vertebral level. The various abdominal fat depots, i.e. visceral fat, subcutaneous fat areas, abdominal deep and superficial subcutaneous fat areas can be appreciated. The fascia (arrows) separating the superficial subcutaneous and deep subcutaneous depots is easily visualized. Despite similar body mass index (BMI) measurements for the male (a), and female (b) subjects, there are significant differences in abdominal fat distribution. BW, body weight; VF, visceral fat; SF, superficial fat; DSF, deep subcutaneous fat; SSF, superficial subcutaneous fat. From reference 18, with permission

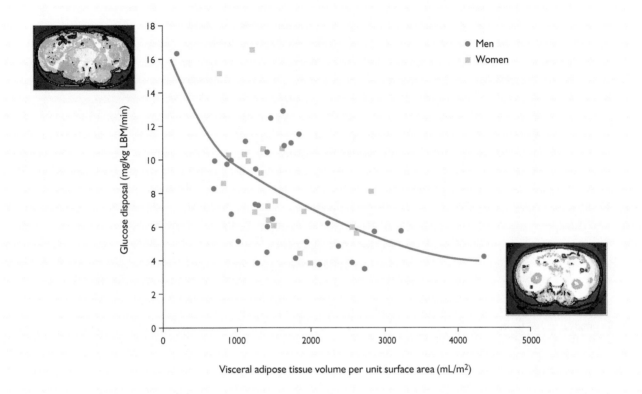

Figure 3.11 Relationship between visceral adipose tissue and skeletal muscle insulin action in both men and women. LBM, lean body mass. From reference 19, with permission

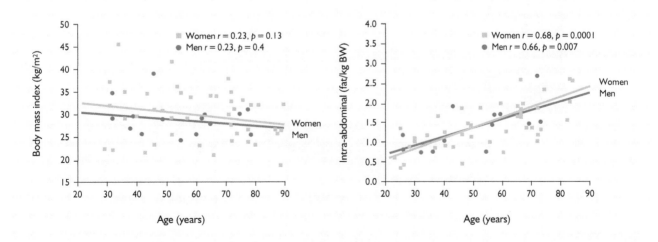

Figure 3.12 Relationship between aging and accumulation of visceral fat. As shown in left panel, this study evaluated both men and women through seven decades. There appeared to be no significant increase in BMI with age for either men or women in this cohort. However, as seen in the right panel, intra-abdominal fat, expressed per kg of body weight, was significantly association with aging in this cohort. The data does suggest redistribution of body fat associated with the aging process. From reference 20 with permission

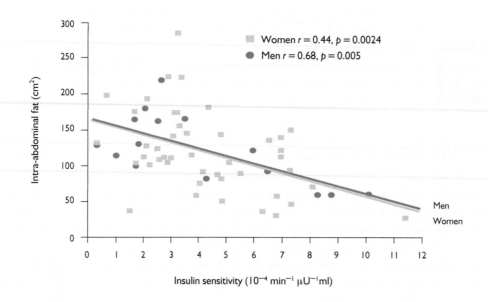

Figure 3.13 Insulin sensitivity is related to intra-abdominal fat accumulation regardless of age or gender. In this study, individuals ranging in age from 20 to 80 years had visceral fat assessed by magnetic resonance imaging and had insulin sensitivity assessed by the modified minimal model. As shown, the greater the visceral fat, the lower the insulin sensitivity. From reference 19, with permission

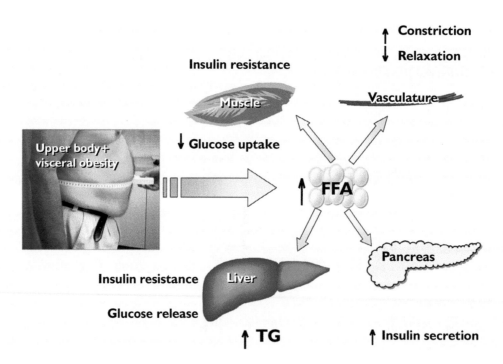

Figure 3.14 Central obesity and insulin resistance are integrally related. There are several possible links between adipose tissue function and insulin resistance determined in other organs such as skeletal muscle or liver. One such link is the regulation of free fatty acid delivery to peripheral tissues. It has been suggested that an expanded adipose tissue mass delivers more free fatty acids to the systemic circulation and to the peripheral tissues. These fatty acids are proposed to compete for substrate utilization in skeletal muscle, which in turn reduces glucose utilization. This increases blood glucose concentration and provides the stimulus for increased insulin secretion and hyperinsulinemia which is a key feature of the insulin-resistance syndrome. Courtesy of Center for Obesity Research and Education

attenuates insulin action has been a topic of great debate. It has also been suggested that the association between abdominal fat and insulin resistance does not prove causality, as it is possible that environmental, biological, or inherited factors that induce insulin resistance also cause abdominal fat accumulation. Nonetheless, it has been proposed that alterations in fatty acid metabolism associated with abdominal obesity may be responsible for the attenuation in insulin action because excessive circulating free fatty acids (FFAs) inhibit the ability of insulin to stimulate muscle glucose uptake and to suppress hepatic glucose production. As such, the notion of a link between abdominal fat, FFA metabolism, and insulin resistance is supported by the observation that basal whole-body FFA flux rates are greater in upper-body obese than in lower-body obese and lean subjects and that diet-induced weight loss decreases whole-body FFA flux

and improves insulin sensitivity (Figures 3.14 and 3.15). Furthermore, the adipose tissue excess, particularly in the visceral compartment, is associated with other co-morbidities including dyslipidemia, hypertension, prothrombotic and proinflammatory states.

Finally, the most recent data regarding the significance of obesity stem from the findings that adipose tissue acts not only as a passive reservoir for energy storage, but also serves as a well known endocrine organ[8]. Specifically, adipose tissue has been shown to express and secrete a number of bioactive proteins referred to as adipocytokines in addition to expressing numerous receptors that allow it to respond to different hormonal signals (Figure 3.16). Thus, in addition to its function to store and release energy, adipose tissue is able to communicate metabolically with other organ systems, and in this way, contributes significantly

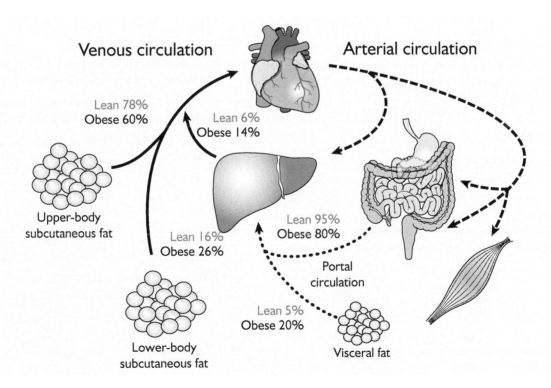

Figure 3.15 It is well established that excessive visceral fat is associated with insulin resistance and other co-morbidities associated with increasing cardiometabolic risk. Furthermore, increased plasma fatty acid concentrations have been postulated to contribute greatly to the metabolic abnormalities associated with abdominal obesity. Visceral fat has been suggested to be more harmful than excess subcutaneous fat, because lipolysis of visceral adipose tissue triglycerides releases free fatty acids (FFAs) into the portal vein, which are then delivered directly to the liver. This schematic demonstrates the approximate relative contributions of FFAs released from lower- and upper-body subcutaneous fat depots and from splanchnic tissues to the systemic venous circulation, and FFAs from visceral fat and the systemic arterial circulation to the portal circulation in lean and obese subjects. From reference 21 with permission

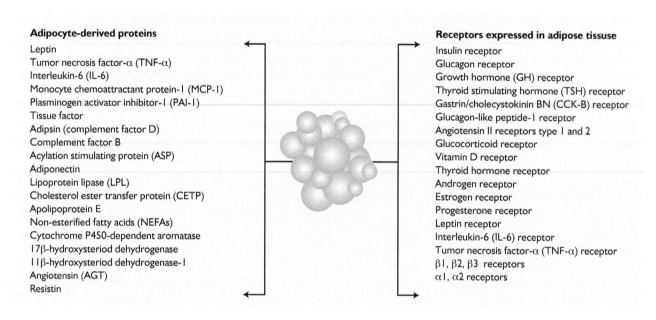

Adipocyte-derived proteins

Leptin
Tumor necrosis factor-α (TNF-α)
Interleukin-6 (IL-6)
Monocyte chemoattractant protein-1 (MCP-1)
Plasminogen activator inhibitor-1 (PAI-1)
Tissue factor
Adipsin (complement factor D)
Complement factor B
Acylation stimulating protein (ASP)
Adiponectin
Lipoprotein lipase (LPL)
Cholesterol ester transfer protein (CETP)
Apolipoprotein E
Non-esterified fatty acids (NEFAs)
Cytochrome P450-dependent aromatase
17β-hydroxysteriod dehydrogenase
11β-hydroxysteriod dehydrogenase-1
Angiotensin (AGT)
Resistin

Receptors expressed in adipose tissuse

Insulin receptor
Glucagon receptor
Growth hormone (GH) receptor
Thyroid stimulating hormone (TSH) receptor
Gastrin/cholecystokinin BN (CCK-B) receptor
Glucagon-like peptide-1 receptor
Angiotensin II receptors type 1 and 2
Glucocorticoid receptor
Vitamin D receptor
Thyroid hormone receptor
Androgen receptor
Estrogen receptor
Progesterone receptor
Leptin receptor
Interleukin-6 (IL-6) receptor
Tumor necrosis factor-α (TNF-α) receptor
β1, β2, β3 receptors
α1, α2 receptors

Figure 3.16   Adipose tissue has been shown to express and secrete a number of bioactive proteins referred to as adipocytokines in addition to expressing numerous receptors that allow it to respond to different hormonal signals. Data from reference 8, with permission

to biological processes that include energy metabolism, neuroendocrine, and immune function[8].

REFERENCES

1. Klein S, Wadden T, Sugerman HJ. AGA technical review on obesity. Gastroenterology 2002; 123: 882–932

2. Troiano RP, Frongillo Jr. EA, Sobal J, Levitsky DA. The relationship between body weight and mortality: a quantitative analysis of combined information from existing studies. Int J Obes Relat Metab Disord 1996; 20: 63–75

3. Calle EE, Thun MJ, Petrelli JM, et al. Body-mass index and mortality in a prospective cohort of US adults. N Engl J Med 1999; 341: 1097–1105

4. Manson JE, Willett WC, Stampfer MJ, et al. Body weight and mortality among women. N Engl J Med 1995; 333: 677–685

5. Smyth S, Heron A. Diabetes and obesity: the twin epidemics. Nat Med 2006; 12: 75–80

6. Flegal KM, Carroll MD, Kuczmarski RJ, Johnson CL. Overweight and obesity in the United States: prevalence and trends, 1960–1994. Int J Obes Relat Metab Disord 1998; 22: 39–47

7. Kahn SE, Prigeon RL, McCulloch DK, et al. Quantification of the relationship between insulin sensitivity and beta-cell function in human subjects. Evidence for a hyperbolic function. Diabetes 1993; 42: 1663–72

8. Kershaw EE, Flier JS. Adipose tissue as an endocrine organ. J Clin Endocrinol Metab 2004; 89: 2548–56

9. Ravussin E, Smith SR. Increased fat intake, impaired fat oxidation, and failure of fat cell proliferation result in ectopic fat storage, insulin resistance, and type 2 diabetes mellitus. Ann NY Acad Sci 2002; 967: 363–78

10. Weyer C, Foley JE, Bogardus C, et al. Enlrged subcutaneous abdominal adipocyte sixe, but not obesity itself, predicts type II diabetes independent of insulin resistance. Diabetologia 2000; 43: 1498–506

11. Despres JP, Lemieux I, Proud'homme D. Treatment of obesity: need to focus on high risk abdominally obese patients. BMJ 2001; 322: 716–20

12. Pi-Sunyer FX. The epidemiology of central fat distribution in relation to disease. Nutr Rev 2004; 62: S120–126

13. Bray GA. An Atlas of Obesity and Weight Control. London: Parthenon Publishing, 2003

14. Rexrode KM, Carey VJ, Hennekens CH, et al. Abdominal adiposity and coronary heart disease in women. JAMA 1998; 280: 1843–8

15. Rexrode KM, Buring JE, Manson JE. Abdominal and total adiposity and risk of coronary heart disease in men. Int J Obes Relat Metab Disord 2001; 25: 1047–56

16. Larsson B. Regional obesity as a health hazard in men – prospective studies. Acta Med Scand Suppl. 1988; 723: 45–51

17. Lean ME, Han TS, Seidell JC. Impairment of health and quality of life in people with large waist circumference. Lancet 1998; 351: 853–6

18. Miyazaki Y, Glass L, Triplitt C, et al. Abdominal fat distribution and peripheral and hepatic insulin resistance in type 2 diabetes mellitus. Am J Physiol Endocrinol Metab 2002; 283: E1135–43

19. Banerji MA, Lebowitz J, Chaiken RL, et al. Relationship of visceral adipose tissue and glucose disposal is independent of sex in black NIDDM subjects. Am J Physiol 1997; 273: E425–32

20. Cefalu WT, Wang ZQ, Werbel S, et al. Contribution of visceral fat mass to the insulin resistance of aging. Metabolism 1995; 44: 954–9

21. Klein S. The case of visceral fat: argument for the defense. J Clin Invest 2004; 113: 1530–2

4 Physiologic systems regulating energy balance, including the endocannabinoid system

It is well established that obesity and insulin resistance are associated with an increased risk for developing type 2 diabetes in addition to developing other cardiometabolic risk factors[1–4]. Fortunately, over the recent past, there has been a rapid and substantive increase in our understanding of the underlying physiologic systems and molecular pathways modulating these conditions. Specifically, key regulators of energy balance and insulin signaling have been elucidated that have aided greatly our understanding of the link between obesity and insulin resistance. As such, the concept of obesity may be simple to grasp in that it develops over time when we take in more calories than we burn, but insight into the mechanisms behind this observation has revealed systems that are complex and highly integrated[5]. Specifically, the epidemic of obesity that is occurring globally indicates the inability of homeostatic mechanisms to offset a sedentary lifestyle and increased caloric intake[6,7]. Furthermore, it is understood that there is a dynamic interplay between the adipose tissue and other key tissues in the body, such as liver, muscle and regulatory centers of the brain. Altered regulation of this integrated and coordinated system inevitably leads to accumulation of body fat, insulin resistance and type 2 diabetes (Figure 4.1). While it is understood that lifestyle intervention is the cornerstone of therapy for obesity, it is also apparent that effective pharmacotherapy, designed to reduce the cardiometabolic risk profile, is urgently needed. In order to develop effective strategies that may modulate molecular mechanisms contributing to obesity and insulin resistance, there must be sound scientific evidence in support of and agreement on the pathogenic mechanisms. This chapter will therefore focus on the physiologic systems and pathways proposed to regulate whole-body energy metabolism and that contribute to or modulate pathways relevant to the development of obesity and/or insulin resistance.

AMP-ACTIVATED PROTEIN KINASE CASCADE

Analogous to the chemicals in an electrical cell or battery, all living cells must continuously maintain a high, non-equilibrium ratio of ATP to ADP to survive. Catabolism charges up the battery by converting ADP and phosphate to ATP, whereas almost all other cellular processes tend to discharge the battery by directly or indirectly converting ATP to ADP and phosphate. The fact that the ATP:ADP ratio in cells usually remains constant indicates that the mechanism that maintains these processes in balance, i.e. the AMPK cascade, is very efficient[9,10]. The AMP-activated protein kinase cascade acts as a metabolic sensor or 'fuel gauge' that monitors cellular AMP and ATP levels because it is activated by increases in the AMP:ATP ratio[11]. Once activated, the enzyme switches off ATP-consuming anabolic pathways and switches on ATP-producing pathways, such as fatty acid oxidation[9–11]. In addition to maintaining the energy status of individual cells, this system plays an important role in whole-body energy balance and it is a key player in the development and treatment of insulin resistance and type 2 diabetes[5,9]. More recent evidence further implicates AMPK as having a pivotal role in energy balance.

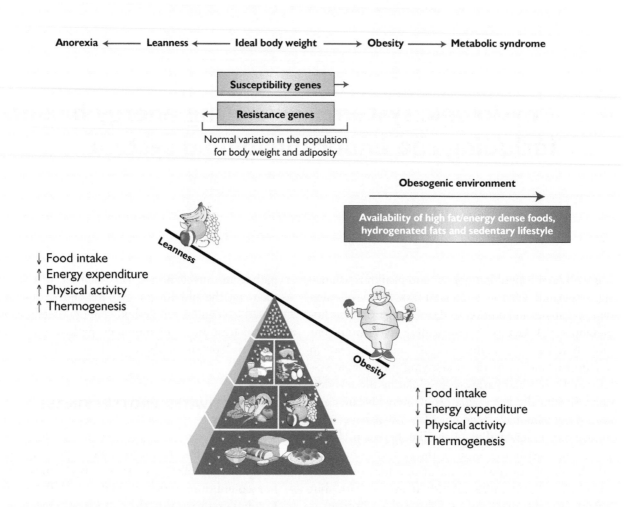

Figure 4.1 The *'Energy Balance Equation'* implies that food consumption, i.e. *'energy intake'*, needs to match energy output, i.e. *'energy expenditure'*, in order to maintain a stable body weight. Major determinants of energy expenditure are: (1) the thermogenic effect of food (TEF), which represents the amount of energy utilized by ingestion and digestion of the food consumed; (2) physical activity; and (3) resting metabolic rate (RMR), determined in large measure by the amount of lean body mass. However, given the many obesity-promoting changes that have occurred in our environment, the whole-body energy balance has shifted toward being overweight and obese in many individuals at an alarming rate. From reference 8, with permission

Specifically, recent animal studies have suggested that AMPK contributes to development of obesity and adipocyte hypertrophy[12]. In addition, several animal studies implicate this system in regulating food intake[13,14]. Thus, it is apparent that the cellular effects of AMPK activation to modulate major pathways of carbohydrate and lipid metabolism and systems regulating whole-body energy balance would be highly beneficial in clinical states of obesity, insulin resistance and type 2 diabetes (Figures 4.2 and 4.3).

LIPOREGULATION

Fat metabolism and carbohydrate metabolism are inherently related. Lipid abnormalities have been shown to have profound effects on carbohydrate metabolism as exemplified by the *'lipotoxicity'* hypothesis. This hypothesis suggests that the abnormal accumulation of lipids, e.g. triglycerides and fatty acyl-CoA in muscle and liver, results in insulin resistance[15,16]. Several lines of evidence support this observation such

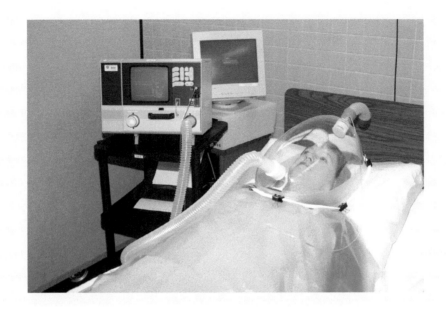

Figure 4.2 Health care professionals typically assess metabolic measurements using indirect calorimetry. With these techniques, resting metabolic rate (RMR) via indirect calorimetry to determine a person's energy expenditure can be determined. RMR via indirect calorimetry is determined by either by oxygen consumption (VO_2) or oxygen consumption and carbon dioxide production (VCO_2). As demonstrated, a subject on an indirect calorimetry machine

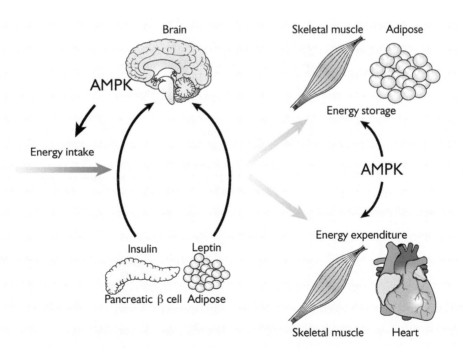

Figure 4.3 Role of AMPK in the regulation of whole body energy metabolism. Energy intake (food) is used for energy expenditure and any excess is stored in the body, e.g. as fat (adipose) or glycogen (liver and skeletal muscles). The hypothalamus plays a key role in the integration of these pathways by hormones, e.g. insulin secreted from pancreatic β-cells and leptin secreted from adipose cells. AMPK inhibits storage pathways and stimulates energy expenditure. In addition, recent studies indicate that activation of AMPK in the hypothalamus increases food intake, whereas inhibition decreases intake. From reference 10, with permission

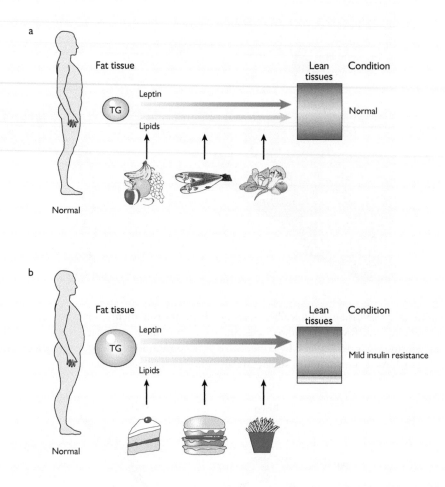

Figure 4.4 A concept of the liporegulatory system and lipid partitioning in normal, healthy subjects. (a) When caloric intake is equal to caloric expenditure, the liporegulatory system is at rest, and the lean tissues contain little or no unmetabolized lipids. (b) During overnutrition, the adipocyte pool expands, and leptin levels rise proportionately. This upregulates oxidative metabolism of long-chain fatty acids in the lean tissues. Thus, ectopic accumulation of surplus lipids is minimal, and partitioning of body fat is well maintained. Nevertheless, there may be modest reduction in insulin sensitivity and glucose tolerance within the normal range. From reference 19, with permission

as studies showing a strong correlation between intramuscular fat content as assessed with nuclear magnetic resonance spectroscopy, and insulin resistance[16,17]. Moreover, insulin sensitivity is restored by treatments that reduce intramuscular lipid accumulation (i.e. low-fat feeding, fasting, and exercise)[18].

When normal and healthy individuals are in energy balance such that caloric intake matches caloric expenditure, their liporegulatory system is at rest[19] (Figure 4.4). When the system is at rest, leptin levels are observed to be low. Leptin is a hormone produced

by adipose tissue and was first known to regulate energy homeostasis by inhibiting food intake and by upregulating energy consumption[20]. More recent findings, however, suggest that leptin is a dual molecule. Not only is it characterized as a hormone involved in energy homeostasis, but increasing evidence also suggests that leptin regulates and participates in both immune homeostasis and inflammatory processes[20]. When an individual chronically consumes more calories than are expended, such that the energy balance equation is altered, adipocytes will expand

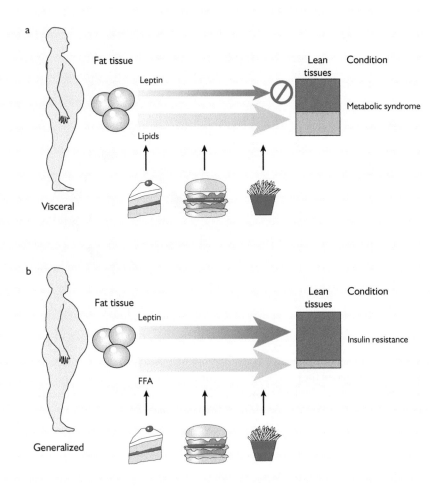

Figure 4.5 Lipid partitioning in diet-induced obesity. (a) Diet-induced visceral obesity is most commonly associated with features consistent with cardiometabolic risk. It is suggested that in visceral obesity, leptin levels, although elevated above those of normal lean subjects, may not be elevated sufficiently to prevent the accumulation of lipids in lean tissues. In addition, there may be resistance to leptin in its target tissues. In any case, the prevalence of obesity and risk factors is greater. (b) In generalized obesity, the hyperleptinemia is greater and is presumably better able to limit ectopic lipid accumulation. Although insulin resistance still occurs, most other features consistent with the metabolic syndrome may be absent. FFA, free fatty acid. From reference 19, with permission

and leptin levels will rise in proportion to the degree of lipid overload[19]. In this context, it is proposed that the elevated leptin level promotes fatty acid oxidation and inhibiting lipogenesis, thereby maintaining the lipid content in the lean tissue at a near-normal level[19] (Figure 4.4).

In clinical conditions associated with abdominal obesity, however, liporegulatory failure may occur in that the circulating level of leptin, although higher than normal, may not be effective and leptin resistance may be observed[20] (Figure 4.5).

ADIPOCYTE DYSFUNCTION AND INSULIN RESISTANCE

Adipose tissue plays a key role in directing whole-body glucose disposal, although it accounts for only about 10% of insulin-stimulated glucose disposal. There is now substantial evidence that factors that regulate adipocyte function can ultimately lead to insulin sensitization in muscle. Along these lines, the discovery of the peroxisome proliferator-activated receptors (PPARs) in the early 1990s has revolutionized

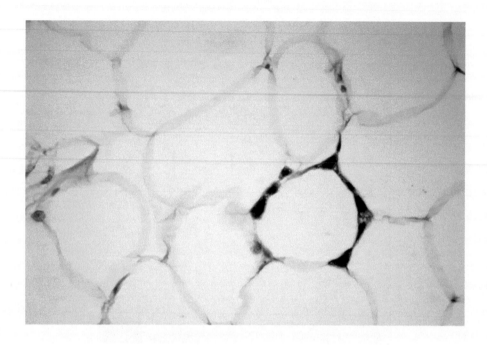

Figure 4.6 CD68+ macrophages in human white adipose tissue. A hypertrophic adipocyte is surrounded by macrophages. Adipose tissue recruits macrophages for reasons that are not entirely clear. However, the local inflammatory milieu is thought to (a) increase adipocyte lipolysis as cytokines downregulate insulin signaling and (b) change the secretion of adipokines such as leptin and adiponectin. Photomicrograph courtesy of Barbara Kozak, PhD

our understanding of fat and carbohydrate metabolism and their interaction. In particular, a large body of evidence has accumulated suggesting that PPARγ is a master regulator in the formation of fat cells and their ability to function normally in the adult[21,22]. PPARγ is induced during adipocyte differentiation and ectopic expression of PPARγ in non-adipogenic cells effectively converts them into mature adipocytes[23,24]. Thus, the discovery and study of the PPARs have contributed greatly to the evidence supporting the role of the adipocyte as having a major effect on skeletal muscle glucose uptake. First, there is evidence that activation of PPARγ in adipose tissue improves its ability to store lipids, thereby reducing 'ectopic' fat storage in liver and muscle[21]. If this metabolic pathway is activated, lipid repartitioning on a whole-body level will occur increasing the triglyceride content of adipose tissue, lowering free fatty acids and triglycerides in the circulation, liver and muscle, resulting in improved insulin sensitivity. In essence, activation of this pathway will improve the 'lipotoxicity' as described for

muscle. Furthermore, adipocytes are derived from pluripotent stem cell precursors and individuals who have a low capacity for proliferation and/or differentiation of precursors into mature fat-storing adipocytes are susceptible to hypertrophy of the existing adipocytes under conditions of energy excess[25]. Thus, adipocyte hypertrophy (i.e. large fat cells) is indicative of a failure to proliferate and/or differentiate, a failure to accommodate an increased energy flux resulting in ectopic (intracellular) storage in sites such as muscle, liver and pancreas, and correlates better with insulin resistance than any other measure of adiposity[26,27] (Figure 4.6).

A second mechanism by which improvement in adipocyte function can improve insulin sensitivity is by altering the release of signaling molecules from fat (adipocytokines) that have metabolic effects in other tissues[27-28]. For example, it is well known that adipocytokines, such as leptin, tumor necrosis factor-α (TNF-α), resistin and adiponectin, have profound metabolic effects. It has been observed that PPARγ

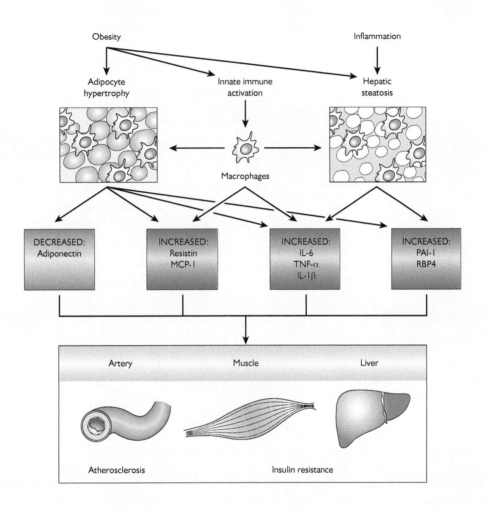

Figure 4.7   The humoral theory of insulin resistance. In this model, insulin resistance results from pathophysiologic levels of circulating factors that are potentially derived from several different cell types. The possible role of adipocytes, macrophages (in adipose tissue, liver and elsewhere), and hepatocytes is shown, along with secreted factors that modulate insulin action at the cellular level. MCP, monocyte chemoattractant protein; IL, interleukin; TNF-α, tumor necrosis factor-α; PAI-1, plasminogen activator inhibitor type 1; RBP, retinol binding protein. From reference 29, with permission

agonists may inhibit the expression of TNF-α and resistin which promote insulin resistance, whereas they may stimulate the production of adiponectin, which promotes fatty acid oxidation and insulin sensitivity in muscle and liver[28] (Figure 4.7). In addition, substantial evidence has accumulated that chronic activation of the proinflammatory pathway in insulin target tissues and in macrophages may underlie the obesity-related component of these insulin-resistant states (Figure 4.8).

ENDOCANNABINOID SYSTEM

A recently characterized physiologic system that plays a major role in modulating energy metabolism is the endocannabinoid–CB$_1$ receptor system (Figure 4.9)[31,32]. The discovery of this system represents a significant advance in understanding mechanisms contributing to the development of obesity and as such, provides targets for new pharmacological approaches to target abdominal obesity and its related metabolic

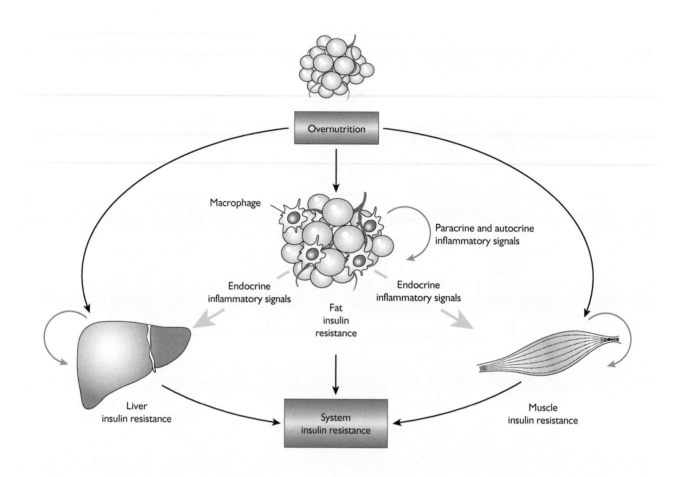

Figure 4.8 The development of systemic insulin resistance in obesity-induced inflammation and stress. In obese states, adipose tissue is under a constant state of metabolic stress, resulting in the activation of the stress and inflammatory response, which leads to the accumulation of macrophages. In this state, adipocytes release cytokines, adipokines and free fatty acids, which can act in a paracrine or autocrine fashion to amplify the proinflammatory state within adipose tissue and cause localized insulin resistance. Adipose tissue also serves as an endocrine organ whereby these cytokines, adipokines and free fatty acids travel to liver and muscle and may decrease insulin sensitivity. In addition to the adipose tissue-derived factors, stress and inflammatory signals can arise independently within liver and muscle, and result in local insulin resistance within these organs. From reference 30, with permission

complications. The endocannabinoid system consists of a family of endogenous agonists that are phospholipid derivatives and locally produced (endocannabinoids) and the receptors which they activate, i.e. $G_{I/O}$-protein-coupled CB_1 receptors[33–35].

It has been reported that the CB_2 receptors are located in key areas of the brain involved in the regulation of appetite/satiety as well as in several tissues/organs such as the autonomic nervous system, the liver, skeletal muscle, gastrointestinal tract and adipose tissue (Figure 4.10)[31,36]. There appears to be

key differences between classic neurotransmitters and the endocannabinoid system as it is now described that endocannabinoids are produced on demand post-synaptically and degraded rapidly (Figure 4.11). There is therefore considerable evidence supporting the notion that the endocannabinoid system has an important role in the regulation of energy balance[37]. For example, it has been demonstrated that the endo-cannabinoid administration increases energy intake and this effect is not observed in animals lacking the CB_1 receptor[38,39]. Furthermore, animals lacking the

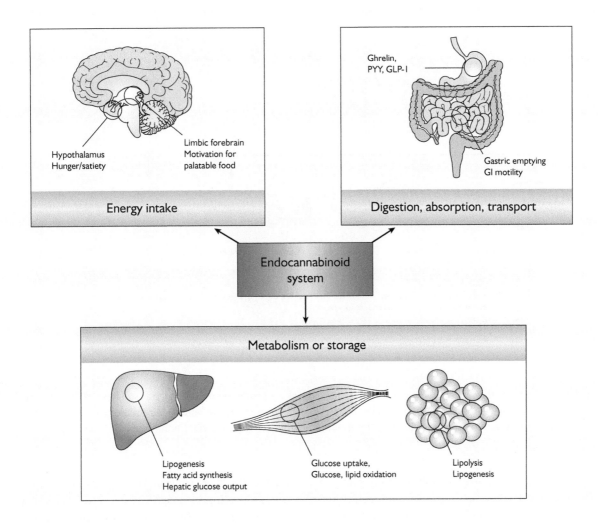

Figure 4.9 The EC system has effects that modulate whole-body energy metabolism. Specifically, the system acts as a major contributor to the energy balance by altering dietary intake. In addition, the system has effects on digestion, absorption, and metabolism of substrates. PYY, peptide YY; GLP-1, glucagon-like protein-1

receptor (knockout mice) are lean and appear to be resistant to diet-induced obesity[32]. Because of these observations, it was postulated that by blocking the CB_1 receptor, this approach would represent an innovative approach for the management of high-risk abdominal obesity and the related cardiometabolic risk[38]. The results from recently completed phase III clinical trials in overweight/ obese patients suggests that this approach may indeed yield substantial clinical benefits[6,40,41].

Rimonabant was the first developed CB_1 blocker. Use of this agent in animals suggested that this drug could induce a reduction in food intake, loss of body weight and body fat, and could improve insulin sensitivity and blood lipids[31,36]. It also appeared that rimonabant could favorably alter the metabolic profile beyond what could be explained by weight loss[32]. The explanation put forth to explain the putative weight-independent effect of the drug appeared to be related to the discovery of the presence of CB_1 receptors on other tissues and organs among which there is adipose tissue[32,42]. It has been suggested that the stimulation of CB_1 receptors in fat cells would promote lipogenesis leading to fat cell hypertrophy[32]. This in turn would reduce production of adiponectin by enlarged adipose cells.

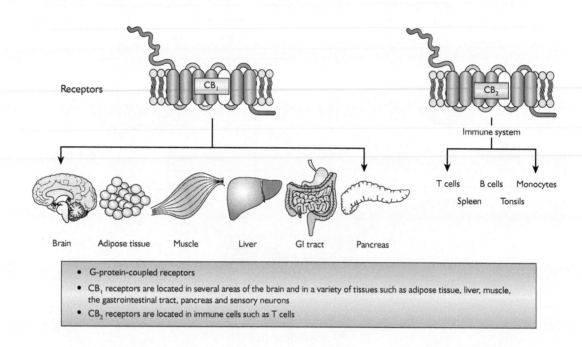

Brain   Adipose tissue   Muscle   Liver   GI tract   Pancreas

- G-protein-coupled receptors
- CB_1 receptors are located in several areas of the brain and in a variety of tissues such as adipose tissue, liver, muscle, the gastrointestinal tract, pancreas and sensory neurons
- CB_2 receptors are located in immune cells such as T cells

Figure 4.10 The cannabinoid (CB) receptors are described as G-protein-coupled receptors. These receptors are located throughout the body, but have particular relevance in that they are present in the brain where major effects may be seen with activation. Endocannabinoids control food intake by modulating the activity of several brain regions

The observations reported in animal studies appear to be quite compatible with the human condition. Specifically, an overstimulation of the endocannabinoid system in human abdominal obesity has been suggested to lead to fat cell hypertrophy and to markedly reduced plasma adiponectin levels, which are well-described features of abdominal obesity[43]. Furthermore, it was reported that the low plasma adiponectin concentration observed in viscerally obese patients was a key factor responsible for their markedly reduced HDL-cholesterol levels[43]. The decreased adiponectin level in subjects with visceral obesity would be postulated to reduce intracellular insulin signaling and therefore induce insulin resistance[44]. This pathway could represent one of the mechanisms by which the overstimulated endocannabinoid system of abdominally obese patients contributes to insulin resistance on a clinical level. In support of this concept are recent data suggesting that an overactivated EC system contributes to fat accumulation in the peripheral tissues such as liver, leading to related metabolic impairments[45–47]. As therefore proposed, CB_1 block-

ade with drugs such as rimonabant will reduce food intake leading to weight loss and to related metabolic improvements. But, it also appears that a weight-loss-independent effect of this drug may be expected from its mechanism of action, likely to be mediated by the blockade of CB_1 receptors located in key systemic metabolic organs/tissues such as the liver and adipose tissue[40] (Figure 4.10).

Rimonabant is currently the first CB_1 receptor blocker under clinical development and the key effects on anthropometric, metabolic and CVD risk variables reported in completed clinical research studies are summarized (Table 4.1). In the first published trial (RIO-Europe), it was reported that treatment with rimonabant for 1 year resulted in a significant weight loss, a substantial reduction in waist circumference and improved metabolic risk factors for diabetes and cardiovascular disease in patients with overall obesity[41]. Specifically, treatment with rimonabant at 20 mg/day reduced fasting insulin, 2-hour plasma insulin, increased HDL-cholesterol concentration and reduced plasma triglyceride levels. It was also suggested

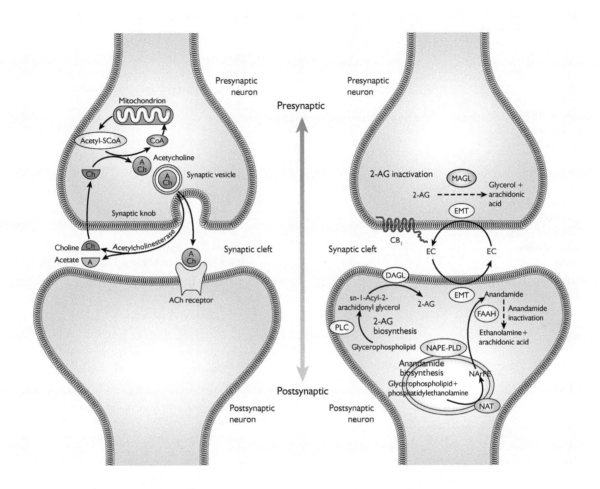

Figure 4.11 Differences between classic neurotransmitters (left) and the endocannabinoid system (ECS) (right). In the classic neurotransmission system, presynaptic release of a neurotransmitter interacts with receptors at the postsynaptic membrane and channels open allowing ions to flow through. This causes a change in the postsynaptic membrane potential. In contrast to this system, endocannabinoids are not stored in vesicles. An action potential triggers the opening of calcium channels and activates the synthesis of endocannabinoids from membrane-bound precursors. The endocannabinoids are released and enter the synaptic cleft. They then bind to the cannabinoid (CB)$_1$ receptor located presynaptically. This reverse pathway is called retrograde signaling. This is important in that the ECS is normally quiet until endocannabinoids are synthesized on demand, taken back up into cells, and degraded. Thus, endocannabinoids act locally. Ach, acetylcholine; DAGL, diacylglycerol lipase; MAGL, monoacylglycerol lipase; 2-AG, 2-arachidonoylglycerol; PLC, phospholipase C; NAT, *N*-acyltransferase; NAPE-PLD, *N*-acylphosphatidyl-ethanolamine-specific phospholipase D; FAAH, fatty acid amide hydrolase; EMT, endocannabinoid membrane transporter; NArPE, *N*-arachindonoyl-phosphatidyl-ethanolamine. Adapted from reference 31, with permission

that 50% of these metabolic effects were independent from the weight loss, suggesting a systemic metabolic effect on CB$_1$ receptors located in peripheral tissues[40].

A second 1-year study was designed to test the effect of rimonabant in dyslipidemic overweight/obese patients (RIO-Lipids). This study also reported that rimonabant therapy at 20 mg/day significantly decreased body weight as well as markedly improving

body composition indicated by a considerable reduction in waist circumference[48]. The weight loss and change in body composition was related to significant improvements in glucose tolerance, reduction in plasma insulin levels, reduction in triglyceride concentrations and increase in HDL-cholesterol levels. An important observation was that the prevalence of patients meeting the NCEP-ATP III criteria for the

Table 4.1 Reported effects of rimonabant on anthropometric, metabolic and cardiovascular disease risk variables

Anthropometric variables
↓ Body weight
↓ Waist circumference

Metabolic and cardiovascular disease risk variables
↓ Triglycerides
↑ HDL-cholestrol
↓ Cholesterol/HDL-cholesterol ratio
↓ Apolipoprotein B/apolipoprotein AI ratio
↑ LDL peak particle size
↓ Proportion of small LDL particles
↑ Proportion of large LDL particles
↑ Insulin sensitivity
↓ Insulin

Improved glucose tolerance
↑ Adiponectin
↓ Leptin
↓ C-reactive protein
↓ Systolic and diastolic blood pressure

LDL, low-density lipoprotein; HDL, high-density lipoprotein

metabolic syndrome was reduced by about 50% among patients treated with rimonabant. In addition, patients treated with rimonabant showed additional improvements in other cardiometabolic risk markers such as favorable effects on LDL particle size and C-reactive protein levels. A low adiponectin concentration was associated with insulin resistance, inflammation and an atherogenic dyslipidemia in the patients prior to treatment with rimonabant. However, plasma adiponectin levels increased by 57% in subjects treated[48]. Therefore, it appears that the favorable improvement of abdominal fat distribution and adiponectin levels are important factors contributing to the effect of CB_1 blockers such as rimonabant on metabolic risk factors for type 2 diabetes and CVD[42]. Thus, rimonabant therapy, by targeting both abdominal obesity and cardiometabolic risk factors in centrally obese patients, provides a novel therapeutic clinical option not previously available.

REFERENCES

1. Wilson PW, D'Agostino RB, Sullivan L, et al. Overweight and obesity as determinants of cardiovascular risk: the Framingham experience. Arch Intern Med 2002; 162: 1867–72

2. Janssen I, Katzmarzyk PT, Ross R. Body mass index, waist circumference, and health risk: evidence in support of current National Institutes of Health guidelines. Arch Intern Med 2002; 162: 2074–9

3. Tuomilehto J, Lindstrom J, Eriksson JG, et al. Prevention of type 2 diabetes mellitus by changes in lifestyle among subjects with impaired glucose tolerance. N Engl J Med 2001; 344: 1343–50

4. Sjöström L, Lindroos AK, Peltonen M, et al. Lifestyle, diabetes, and cardiovascular risk factors 10 years after bariatric surgery. N Engl J Med 2004; 351: 2683–93

5. Evans RM, Barish GD, Wang YU. PPARs and the complex journey to obesity. Nat Med 2004; 10: 355–61

6. Despres JP, Golay A, Sjostrom L; Rimonabant in Obesity-Lipids Study Group. Effects of rimonabant on metabolic risk factors in overweight patients with dyslipidemia. N Engl J Med 2005; 353: 2121–34

7. Flier JS. Obesity wars: molecular progress confronts an expanding epidemic. Cell 2004; 116: 337–50

8. Cefalu WT, Greenway F. Pharmacologic agents and nutritional supplements in the treatment of obesity. In Fonseca VA, ed. Clinical Diabetes: Translating Research into Practice. Philadelphia, PA: Elsevier, 2006

9. Hardie DG. Minireview: the AMP-activated protein kinase cascade: the key sensor in cellular energy status. Endocrinology 2003; 144: 5179–83

10. Fryer LGD, Carling D. AMP-activated protein kinase and the metabolic syndrome. Biochem Soc Trans 2005; 33: 362–6

11. Hardie DG, Carling D, Carlson M. The AMP-activated/snf1 protein kinase subfamily: metabolic sensors of the eukaryotic cell? Ann Rev Biochem 1998; 67: 821–55

12. Villena JA, Viollet B, Andreelli F, et al. Induced adiposity and adipocyte hypertrophy in mice lacking the AMP-activated protein kinase-α2 subunit. Diabetes 2004; 53: 2242–9

13. Minokoshi Y, Alquier T, Furukawa N, et al. AMP-kinase regulates food intake by responding to hormonal and nutrient signals in the hypothalamus. Nature 2004; 428: 569–74

14. Andersson U, Filipsson K, Abbott CR, et al. AMP-activated protein kinase plays a role in the control of food intake. J Biol Chem 2004; 26; 279: 12005–8

15. Perseghin G, Scifo P, De Cobelli F, et al. Intramyocellular triglyceride content is a determinant of in vivo insulin resistance in humans: a 1H-13C nuclear mag-

netic resonance spectroscopy assessment in offspring of type 2 diabetic parents. Diabetes 1999; 48: 1600–6

16. McGarry JD. Banting lecture 2001: dysregulation of fatty acid metabolism in the etiology of type 2 diabetes. Diabetes 2002; 51: 7–18

17. Dresner A, Laurent D, Marcucci M, et al. Effects of free fatty acids on glucose transport and IRS-1 associated phosphatidylinositol 3-kinase activity. J Clin Invest 1999; 103: 253–9

18. Ellis BA, Poynten A, Lowy AJ, et al. Long-chain acyl-CoA esters as indicators of lipid metabolism and insulin sensitivity in rat and human muscle. Am J Physiol Endocrinol Metab 2000; 279: E554–60

19. Unger RH. Minireview: weapons of lean body mass destruction: the role of ectopic lipids in the metabolic syndrome. Endocrinology 2003; 144: 5159–65

20. Otero M, Lago R, Gomz R, et al. Leptin: a metabolic hormone that functions like a proinflammatory adipokine. Drug News Perspect 2006; 19: 21–6

21. Shulman GI. Cellular mechanisms of insulin resistance. J Clin Invest 2000; 106: 171–6

22. Tontonoz P, Hu E, Spiegelman BM. Stimulation of adipogenesis in fibroblasts by PPAR γ2, a lipid-activated transcription factor. Cell 1994; 79: 1147–56

23. Rosen ED, Sarraf P, Troy AE, et al. PPARγ is required for the differentiation of adipose tissue in vivo and in vitro. Mol Cell 1999; 4: 611–17

24. Ravussin E, Smith SR. Increased fat intake, impaired fat oxidation, and failure of fat cell proliferation result in ectopic fat storage, insulin resistance, and type 2 diabetes mellitus. Ann NY Acad Sci 2002; 967: 363–78

25. Weyer C, Foley JE, Bogardus C, et al. Enlarged subcutaneous abdominal adipocyte size, but not obesity itself, predicts type II diabetes independent of insulin resistance. Diabetologia 2000; 43: 1498–506

26. Steppan CM, Bailey ST, Bhat S, et al. The hormone resistin links obesity to diabetes. Nature 2001; 409: 307–12

27. Ferre P. The biology of peroxisome proliferator-activated receptors: relationship with lipid metabolism and insulin sensitivity. Diabetes 2004; 53 (Suppl 1): S43–50

28. Havel PJ. Update on adipocyte hormones: regulation of energy balance and carbohydrate/lipid metabolism. Diabetes 2004; 53 (Suppl 1): S143–51

29. Lazar MA. The humoral side of insulin resistance. Nat Med 2006; 12: 43–4

30. de Luca C, Olefsky J. Stressed out about obesity and insulin resistance. Nat Med 2006; 12: 41–2

31. Di Marzo V, Bifulco M, De Petrocellis L. The endocannabinoid system and its therapeutic exploitation. Nat Rev Drug Discov 2004; 3: 771–84

32. Cota D, Marsicano G, Tschop M, et al. The endogenous cannabinoid system affects energy balance via central orexigenic drive and peripheral lipogenesis. J Clin Invest 2003; 112: 423–31

33. Devane WA, Hanus L, Breuer A, et al. Isolation and structure of a brain constituent that binds to the cannabinoid receptor. Science 1992; 258: 1946–9

34. Hanus L, Abu-Lafi S, Fride E, et al. 2-Arachidonyl glyceryl ether, an endogenous agonist of the cannabinoid CB1 receptor. Proc Natl Acad Sci USA 2001; 98: 3662–5

35. Howlett AC, Barth F, Bonner TI, et al. International Union of Pharmacology. XXVII. Classification of cannabinoid receptors. Pharmacol Rev 2002; 54: 161–202

36. Pagotto U, Pasquali R. Fighting obesity and associated risk factors by antagonising cannabinoid type 1 receptors. Lancet 2005; 365: 1363–4

37. Di Marzo V, Matias I. Endocannabinoid control of food intake and energy balance. Nat Neurosci 2005; 8: 585–9

38. Sugiura T, Kondo S, Sukagawa A, et al. 2-Arachidonoylglycerol: a possible endogenous cannabinoid receptor ligand in brain. Biochem Biophys Res Commun 1995; 215: 89–97

39. Gaoni Y, Mechoulam R. Hashish III: isolation, structure and partial synthesis of an active constituent of hashish. J Am Chem Soc 1964; 86: 1646–7

40. Després J-P, Lemieux I, Alméras N. Contribution of CB1 blockade to the management of high-risk abdominal obesity. Part II: The Endocannabinoids and Regulation of Energy Balance; The Endocannabinoid System: a Target for Anti-Obesity Drugs. Int J Obes 2006; 30: S44–52

41. Van Gaal LF, Rissanen AM, Scheen AJ, et al. Effects of the cannabinoid-1 receptor blocker rimonabant on weight reduction and cardiovascular risk factors in overweight patients: 1-year experience from the RIO-Europe study. Lancet 2005; 365: 1389–97

42. Pertwee RG. Pharmacology of cannabinoid CB1 and CB2 receptors. Pharmacol Ther 1997; 74: 129–80

43. Côté M, Mauriège P, Bergeron J, et al. Adiponectinemia in visceral obesity: impact on glucose tolerance and plasma lipoprotein and lipid levels in men. J Clin Endocrinol Metab 2005; 90: 1434–9

44. Trujillo ME, Scherer PE. Adiponectin – journey from an adipocyte secretory protein to biomarker of the metabolic syndrome. J Intern Med 2005; 257: 167–75

45. Marchesini G, Brizi M, Bianchi G, et al. Nonalcoholic fatty liver disease: a feature of the metabolic syndrome. Diabetes 2001; 50: 1844–50

46. Banerji MA, Buckley MC, Chaiken RL, et al. Liver fat, serum triglycerides and visceral adipose tissue in insulin-sensitive and insulin-resistant black men with NIDDM. Int J Obes Relat Metab Disord 1995; 19: 846–50

47. Nguyen-Duy TB, Nichaman MZ, et al. Visceral fat and liver fat are independent predictors of metabolic risk factors in men. Am J Physiol Endocrinol Metab 2003; 284: E1065–71

48. Després JP, Golay A, Sjöström L, Rimonabant in Obesity-Lipids Study Group. Effects of rimonabant on metabolic risk factors in overweight patients with dyslipidemia. N Engl J Med 2005; 353: 2121–34

5 Traditional metabolic risk factors

HYPERGLYCEMIA

Subjects with the metabolic syndrome have insulin resistance as a core feature, which results in impaired glucose tolerance or frank hyperglycemia.

Epidemiological studies have shown that patients with diabetes mellitus and glucose intolerance are at increased risk for coronary heart disease (CHD). In the first 20 years of the Framingham Heart Study, the incidence of cardiovascular disease among men with diabetes was twice that among men without diabetes, and among women with diabetes the incidence of cardiovascular disease was three times that among women without diabetes[1]. Also, in the Framingham Offspring Study, compared with normal glucose tolerance, subjects with impaired glucose tolerance or an impaired fasting glucose were more likely, and those with diabetes were significantly more likely, to have subclinical coronary atherosclerosis.

The 10-year follow-up of the Munich General Practitioner Project was a prospective study evaluating factors predicting macrovascular disease and overall mortality in non-insulin-dependent diabetic (NIDDM) patients. In a univariate analysis, those who died from macrovascular causes had significantly higher fasting blood glucose and hemoglobin (Hb)A1c levels. After adjustment for traditional risk factors, HbA1c remained an independent predictor of macrovascular disease[2]. In the prospective EPIC-Norfolk study, HbA1c concentrations predicted all cause, cardiovascular, ischemic heart disease, and non-cardiovascular mortality independent of age and known risk factors. When diabetes status and HbA1c concentration were both included in the same model, diabetes was no longer a significant independent predictor of mortality. An increase of 1% in HbA1c concentration was associated with roughly a 40% increase in cardiovascular or ischemic heart disease mortality. After a history of diabetes or those with a HbA1c concentration of > 7%, and those with a prior history of heart disease and stroke were excluded, the relative risk of all cause mortality for a 1% increase in HbA1c was 1.46 (1.00–2.12, $p = 0.05$) adjusted for age and risk factors (Figure 5.1)[3]. Taken together these data suggest that glycemia itself is an important risk factor for adverse cardiovascular events. The beneficial effect of glycemic control on cardiovascular outcomes was suggested by early intervention trials which showed that reducing glucose with oral hypoglycemics provided cardioprotection .

Recently two important studies have shed further light on the importance of more intensive glycemic control[4,5]. The Diabetes Control and Complications Trial (DCCT) demonstrated that among patients with type 1 diabetes mellitus, compared with conventional treatment, intensive control of hyperglycemia with insulin reduced the risk of any cardiovascular disease outcome by 42% (Figure 5.2) and the risk of non-fatal myocardial infarction, stroke, or death from cardiovascular disease by 57%[4]. Similarly the PROspective pioglitAzone Clinical Trial In macroVascular Events (PROACTIVE) which assessed the benefit of pioglitazone versus placebo in patients with type 2 diabetes mellitus and vascular disease demonstrated that pioglitazone reduced the risk of macrovascular complications by 16% over 3 years (Figure 5.3)[5].

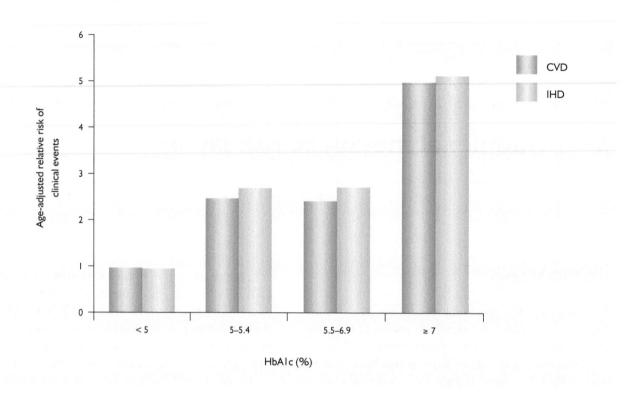

Figure 5.1 Age-adjusted risk of cardiovascular disease (CVD) and ischemic heart disease (IHD) by glycosylated hemoglobin (HbA1c) concentration in men aged 45–79 years from the EPIC-Norfolk study. The risk of clinical events rose with increasing HbA1c levels and was lowest in those with <5% HbA1c, which is below the cut-off for a normal HbA1c. From reference 3, with permission

The exact mechanism by which hyperglycemia increases cardiovascular risk is unclear. Several mechanisms have been proposed (Figure 5.4) including glycation of circulating proteins which leads to the production of advanced glycation end products (AGE) which are associated with increased clinical risk (Figure 5.5)[6] and also have a number of diverse biological effects (Figure 5.6). Glycation of circulating lipoproteins also increases the atherogenicity of LDL cholesterol and thus may contribute to accelerated atherosclerosis. Direct effects of glucose on the vessel wall may also contribute to endothelial activation, resulting in increased expression of adhesion molecules, reduced production of tissue plasminogen activator (tPA), and increased production of plasminogen activator inhibitor (PAI-1) leading to a hypofibrinolytic state and inflammation. Finally, hyperglycemia may contribute to increased left ventricular (LV) stiffness and renal dysfunction which are both independent predictors of clinical risk.

HIGH-DENSITY LIPOPROTEIN CHOLESTEROL

The earliest histological lesion of atherosclerosis is the fatty streak (Figure 5.7)[7] which comprises of lipid-rich 'foam cells' derived from smooth muscle cells which have migrated from the media and from macrophages which originate as blood monocytes. Over time these progress to a severe flow limiting stenosis (Figure 5.8)[8] consisting of multilayered fibroatheroma (Figure 5.9)[8].

The key role of high-density lipoprotein (HDL) as a carrier of excess cellular cholesterol in the reverse cholesterol transport pathway is believed to provide protection against atherosclerosis. In reverse cholesterol transport, peripheral tissues (e.g. vessel-wall macrophages) remove their excess cholesterol through the ATP-binding cassette transporter 1 (ABCA1) to poorly lipidated apolipoprotein A-I, forming

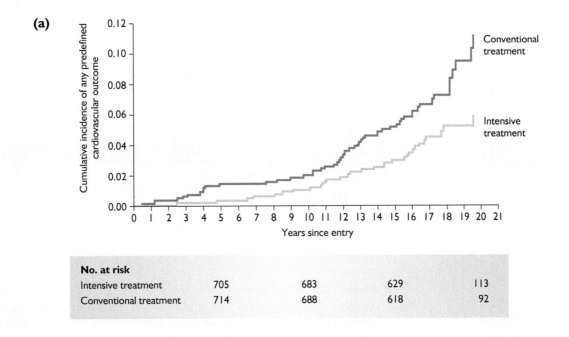

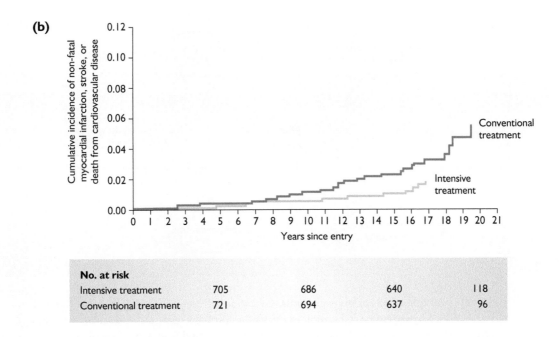

Figure 5.2 Data from the Diabetes Control and Complications Trial (DCCT) showing the cumulative incidence of any cardiovascular disease outcome (a) and of the first occurrence of non-fatal myocardial infarction, stroke, or death from cardiovascular disease (b) among patients with type 1 diabetes mellitus. Compared with conventional treatment, intensive control of hyperglycemia with insulin reduced the risk of any cardiovascular disease outcome by 42% ($p = 0.02$) (a) and reduced the risk of the first occurrence of non-fatal myocardial infarction, stroke, or death from cardiovascular disease by 57% ($p = 0.02$) (b). From reference 4, with permission

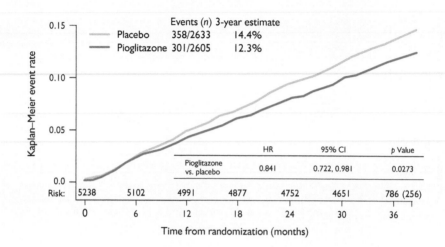

Figure 5.3 Data from the PROspective pioglitAzone Clinical Trial In macroVascular Events (PROACTIVE) which assessed the benefit of pioglitazone vs. placebo in addition to standard care of patients with type 2 diabetes mellitus. Pioglitazone improved glycemic control by an absolute value of 0.8% and reduced the risk of macrovascular complications by 16% over 3 years. From reference 5, with permission

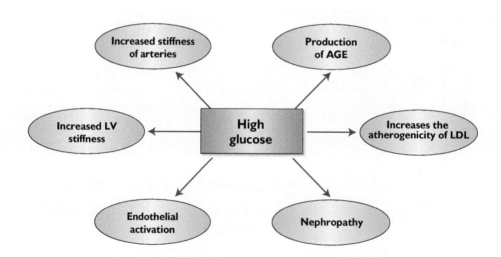

Figure 5.4 Schematic of the multiple effects of hyperglycemia. Glycation of collagen leads to increased arterial stiffness and may contribute to increased risk of hypertension. Glycation of circulating proteins leads to the production of advanced glycation end products (AGE), which have a number of deleterious effects on the vessel wall. Glycation of circulating lipoproteins increases the atherogenicity of LDL cholesterol and oxidized LDL. This leads to accelerated atherosclerosis and increased endothelial cell apoptosis increasing the risk of thrombosis. Glycation of the renal microvasculature results in progressive deterioration in renal function and contributes to increased cardiovascular risk. Direct effects of glucose on the endothelium contribute to endothelial activation, resulting in increased expression of adhesion molecules, reduced production of tissue plasminogen activator (tPA), and increased production of plasminogen activator inhibitor (PAI-1) leading to hypofibrinolysis and inflammatory cell accumulation. Finally, hyperglycemia may contribute to increased left ventricular (LV) stiffness and diastolic dysfunction

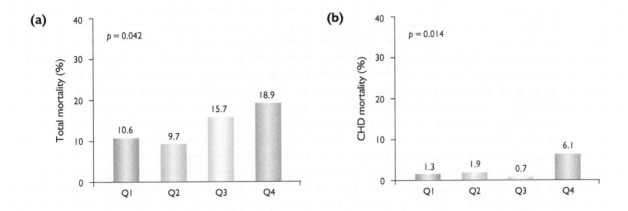

Figure 5.5 Adjusted risk of total (a) and CHD (b) mortality among non-diabetic women by quartiles of plasma AGE (advanced glycation end products). Quartile 4 was associated with a higher risk of total and CHD mortality compared with quartiles 1–3, even after adjusting for age, body mass index (BMI), hypertension, smoking, total cholesterol, HDL cholesterol, and triglycerides. From reference 6, with permission

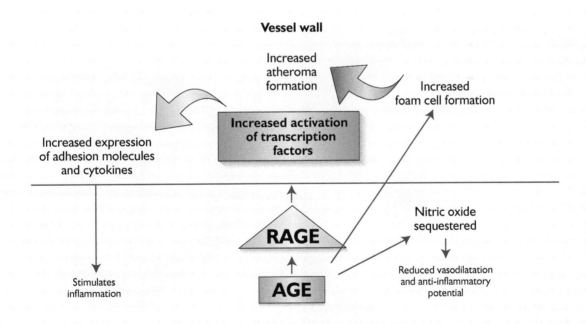

Figure 5.6 Schematic of the biological effects of advanced glycation end products (AGE) at the vessel wall. AGE are the short- and long-term modification products of glycation or glycoxidation of proteins and lipids and have been linked to premature atherosclerosis in diabetic patients as well as in non-diabetic subjects. AGE are a heterogeneous group of compounds that have multiple biological effects, some of which are mediated by interacting with receptors, including the receptor for AGE (RAGE), on endothelial cells, smooth muscle cells, and macrophages. AGE may contribute to the development of atherosclerosis by activating the transcription factor nuclear factor kB (NF-kB) through RAGE binding, resulting in induction of cellular adhesion molecule expression and cytokine activation, thus driving inflammation in the vessel wall. Glycoxidation of lipoproteins increases foam cell formation. AGE also sequestrate NO and mediate impaired endothelial function. Increased AGE modification of long-lived proteins, such as collagen, increases cross-linking and stiffening of arteries

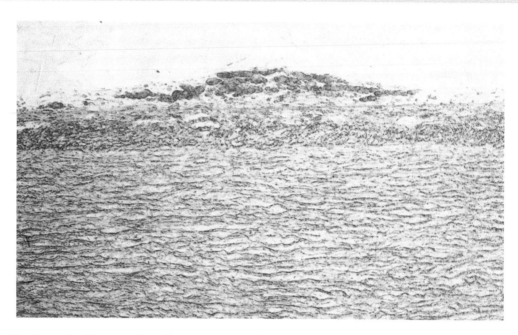

Figure 5.7 Histology of a fatty streak in the intima of the human aorta. The raised area comprises lipid-rich 'foam cells' derived from smooth muscle cells which have migrated from the media and from macrophages which originate as blood monocytes. Fat is stained red with oil red O. From reference 7, with permission

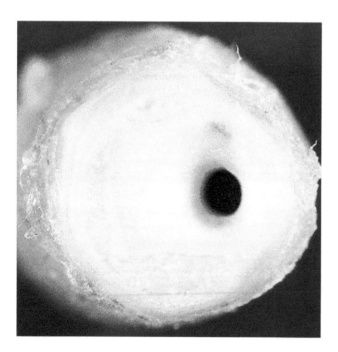

Figure 5.8 Cross-section of anterior descending coronary artery, greatly narrowed by a lipid-rich lesion about 3.5 cm beyond the main bifurcation, viewed here before processing for histology. From a 40-year-old man whose sudden and unexpected death was due to myocardial infarction. From Stary HC. Atlas of Atherosclerosis: Progression and Regression, 2nd edn. Lancaster, UK: Parthenon Publishing, 2003: 104 (reference 8), with permission

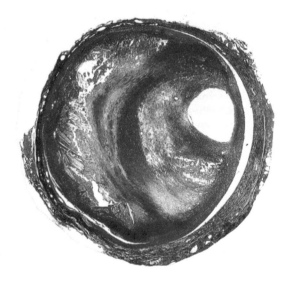

Figure 5.9 Multilayered fibroatheroma in a coronary artery cross-section made 0.5 cm distal to that in Figure 5.8. There are two lipid cores and two thick fibromuscular layers, with one set of core and fibromuscular layer stacked upon the other set. Lesions which severely obstruct the vessel lumen even without superimposed thrombosis (as here) are found in severe hyperlipidemia. From Stary HC. Atlas of Atherosclerosis: Progression and Regression, 2nd edn. Lancaster, UK: Parthenon Publishing, 2003: 104 (reference 8), with permission

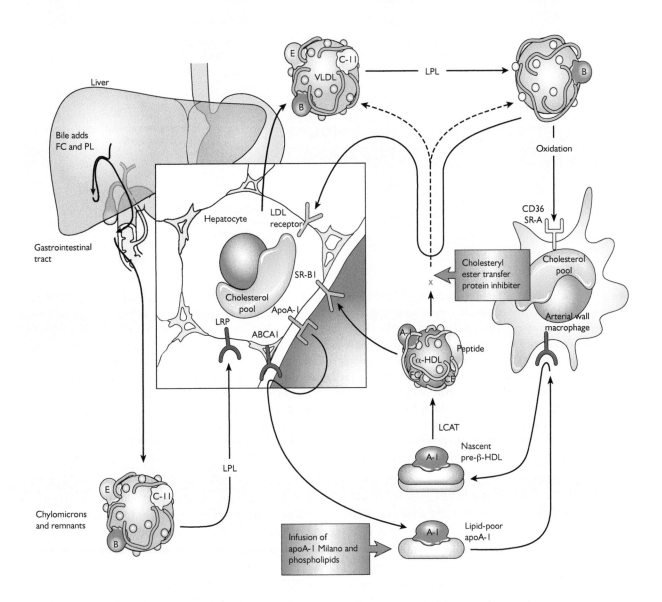

Figure 5.10 Schematic of the reverse cholesterol transport pathway. In reverse cholesterol transport, lipid-poor pre-β-HDL cholesterol, rich in apolipoprotein A-I (ApoA-I), is synthesized by the liver or intestinal mucosa and released into the circulation. There it promotes the transfer of excess cellular-free cholesterol (FC) from macrophages to ApoA-I by interacting with the ATP-binding cassette transporter A1 (ABCA1) in arterial-wall macrophages. Plasma lecithin-cholesterol acyltransferase (LCAT) converts free cholesterol in pre-β-HDL cholesterol to cholesteryl ester (CE), resulting in the maturation of pre-β-HDL cholesterol to mature α-HDL cholesterol. α-HDL cholesterol is transported to the liver by a direct or indirect pathway. In the direct pathway, selective uptake of cholesteryl ester by hepatocytes occurs with the scavenger receptor, class B, type 1 (SR-B1). In the indirect pathway, HDL cholesterol cholesteryl ester is exchanged for triglycerides (TG) in apolipoprotein B-rich particles (B), LDL cholesterol, and very-low-density lipoprotein (VLDL) cholesterol through cholesteryl ester-transfer protein (CETP), with uptake of cholesteryl ester by the liver through the LDL receptor (LDLR). Cholesterol that is returned to the liver is secreted as bile acids and cholesterol. Acquired triglycerides in the modified HDL cholesterol particle are subjected to hydrolysis by hepatic lipase (HL), thereby regenerating small HDL cholesterol particles and pre-β-HDL cholesterol for participation in reverse cholesterol transport. PL, plasma lecithin; E, apolipoprotein-E-rich particles. From reference 9, with permission

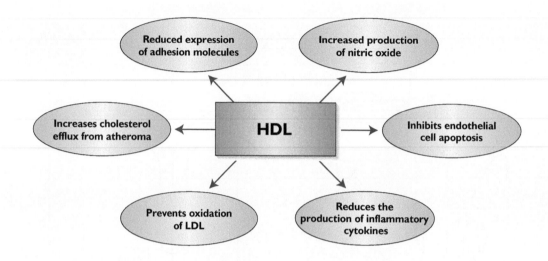

Figure 5.11 Schematic of beneficial effects of HDL. Several studies have shown that HDL improves endothelial function. HDL attenuates expression of adhesion molecules such as vascular intracellular adhesion molecule-1 (VCAM-1) and E-selectin, as well as inflammatory cytokines such as interleukin (IL)-8 that promote leukocyte extravasation into the vessel wall. Infusion of HDL has been shown to increase nitric oxide synthetase activity and therefore nitric oxide bioavailability, which promotes vasodilatation. Other studies have shown that HDL inhibits endothelial apoptosis by the inhibition of typical apoptosis pathways, such as the activation of caspases, and activates protein kinase Akt, a mediator of antiapoptotic signaling. A growing body of evidence suggests that HDL exerts part of its antiatherogenic effect by counteracting LDL oxidation. HDL inhibits the oxidation of LDL and the formation of lipid hydroperoxides. Inhibition of LDL oxidation by HDL is also attributed to the high content of antioxidants in HDL such as apoA-I and to the presence of several enzymes, such as paraoxonase, platelet activating factor acetylhydrolase, and glutathione peroxidase, which prevent LDL oxidation or degrade its bioactive products

pre-α-HDL. HDL consists of a heterogeneous class of lipoproteins containing approximately equal amounts of lipid and protein (Figure 5.10)[9]. The various HDL subclasses vary in quantitative and qualitative content of lipids, apolipoproteins, enzymes, and lipid transfer proteins, resulting in differences in shape, density, size, charge, and antigenicity. Beyond reverse cholesterol transport HDL is believed to have other beneficial effects including improving endothelial function (Figure 5.11). HDL also attenuates expression of adhesion molecules and inflammatory cytokines which promote leukocyte extravasation into the vessel wall. Infusion of HDL has been shown to increase nitric oxide synthetase activity promoting vasodilatation. HDL also inhibits the oxidation of LDL and the formation of lipid hydroperoxides which reduce inflammation. Sujects with metabolic syndrome have low levels of HDL which is believed to contribute to their cardiometabolic risk. The biological effects of HDL are diverse (Figure 5.11) and in addition to

reverse cholesterol transport, antioxidant and anti inflammatory effects are likely to be important.

A large number of prospective observational studies have generally reported inverse associations between HDL cholesterol concentrations and the risk of CHD[10–15], with the largest study reporting that a 1 mg/dL increase in HDL cholesterol is associated with a CHD decrease of 2% in men and 3% in women[10]. Furthermore, the association of HDL cholesterol is proportionally about 50% stronger in women than in men[10]. In the Honolulu Heart Study (Figure 5.12) the age-adjusted incidence of atherosclerotic events was higher in subjects with a low HDL at every level of total cholesterol[16]. Among subjects with established coronary disease the highest event rates were observed among those with a HDL-C below 28 mg/dL and lowest among those with a HDL above 50 mg/dL (Figure 5.13)[17]. The American National Cholesterol Education Program considers HDL cholesterol to be an optional secondary target of lipid treatment[18], whereas the

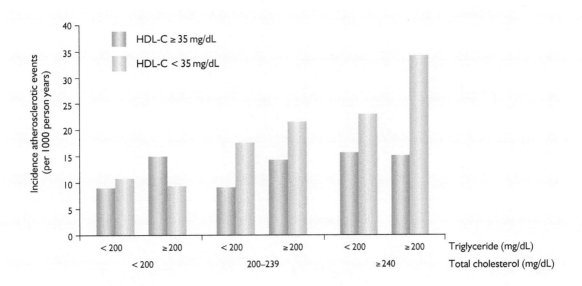

Figure 5.12 Data from the Honolulu Heart Study demonstrating the age-adjusted incidence of atherosclerotic events per 1000 person years by HDL cholesterol (HDL-C), triglyceride, and total cholesterol levels (between 1970 and 1988). At every level of total cholesterol, subjects with a low HDL are at increased risk of atherosclerotic events. From reference 16, with permission

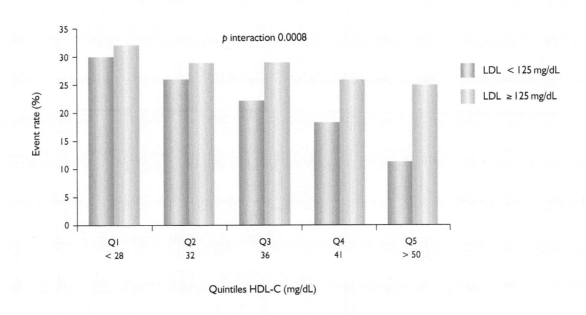

Figure 5.13 Data from the CARE trial showing coronary event rates according to baseline HDL-C concentrations in participants with baseline LDL < 125 or ≥ 125 mg/dL assigned to placebo. Median concentrations (mg/dL) are shown for each quintile of HDL-C. The event rates were highest in those with a HDL-C below 28 mg/dL and lowest among those with a HDL above 50 mg/dL. Note that all patients had a history of coronary artery disease. From reference 17, with permission

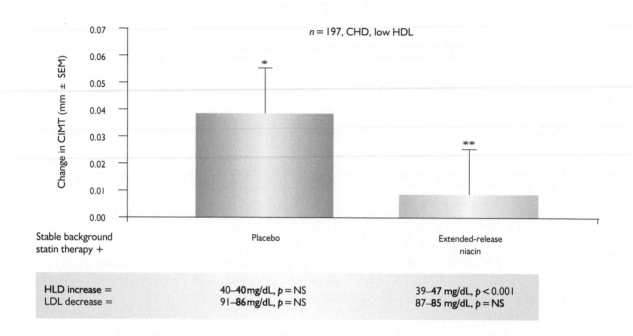

Figure 5.14 Using assessment of carotid intima media thickness (CIMT), which is a surrogate of CV risk, has shown that raising HDL has a significant effect on retarding the progression of atherosclerosis. Data reference 21, with permission. *$p<0.001$; **$p=0.23$

European Consensus Panel recommend a minimum target for HDL of 1.03 mmol/L in certain patients such as diabetics[19].A variety of studies using fibrates have assessed the relative merit of raising HDL or niacin. A recent meta-analysis of these data suggests that there is a 2.5% reduction in CHD events for every 1% rise in HDL cholesterol with fibrates and a 1.7% reduction for every 1% rise in HDL cholesterol with niacin[20]. In addition there is now direct evidence of a beneficial effect of niacin on the atherosclerotic process itself, as niacin reduces the progression of carotid intima media thickness (CIMT) (Figure 5.14)[21].

ATHEROGENIC DYSLIPIDEMIA

Insulin resistant states such as the metabolic syndrome are commonly associated with an atherogenic dyslipidemia that contributes to significantly higher risk of atherosclerosis and cardiovascular disease. Emerging evidence suggests that insulin resistance and its associated metabolic dyslipidemia result from perturbations in key molecules of the insulin signaling pathway, including overexpression of key phosphatases, and downregulation and/or activation of key protein kinase cascades, leading to a state of mixed hepatic insulin resistance and sensitivity. These signaling changes in turn cause an increased expression of sterol regulatory element binding protein (SREBP) 1c, induction of *de novo* lipogenesis, and higher activity of microsomal triglyceride transfer protein (MTP), which together with high exogenous free fatty acid (FFA) flux collectively stimulate the hepatic production of apolipoprotein B (apoB)-containing very-low-density lipoprotein (VLDL) particles (Figure 5.15). When VLDL and triglyceride (TG) levels are high there is enhanced transfer of TG to LDL and HDL making these triglyceride rich and the reverse transport of cholesteryl ester into VLDL occurs (Figure 5.16). Subsequently, VLDL is broken down into small atherogenic remnant particles and the triglyceride-rich LDL is broken down by hepatic lipase into small dense LDL. The TG-rich HDL are broken down into small dense HDL which are easily cleared from the circulation reducing the amount of HDL available for reverse cholesterol transport. VLDL overproduction underlies

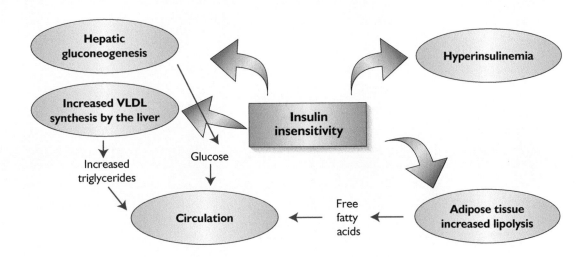

Figure 5.15 Schematic of the most fundamental defect in patients with metabolic syndrome which is resistance to the cellular actions of insulin, particularly resistance to insulin-stimulated glucose uptake. Insulin insensitivity appears to cause hyperinsulinemia, enhanced hepatic gluconeogenesis and increased glucose output. Reduced suppression of lipolysis in adipose tissue leads to a high free fatty acid flux, and increased hepatic very-low-density lipoprotein (VLDL) secretion causing hypertriglyceridemia and reduced plasma levels of high-density lipoprotein (HDL) cholesterol

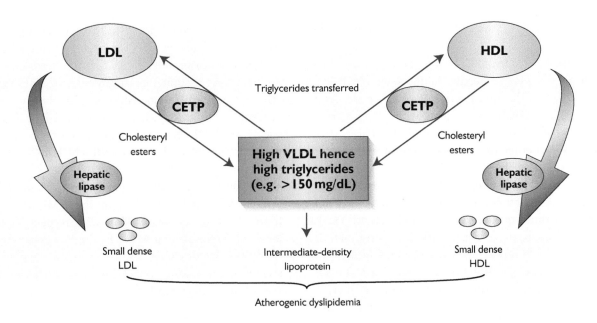

Figure 5.16 Schematic showing the consequences of hypertriglyceridemia and the genesis of atherogeneic dyslipidemia. When VLDL and hence triglyceride (TG) levels are high there is enhanced transfer of TG to LDL and HDL making these triglyceride rich, while there is reverse transport of cholesteryl estr into VLDL. Subsequently, VLDL is broken down into small atherogenic remnant particles like intermediate-density lipoprotein (IDL). the triglyceride-rich LDL is broken down by hepatic lipase into small dense LDL. The TG-rich HDL are broken down into small dense HDL which are easily cleared from the circulation reducing the amount of HDL available for reverse cholesterol transport. CETP, cholesteryl ester-transfer protein

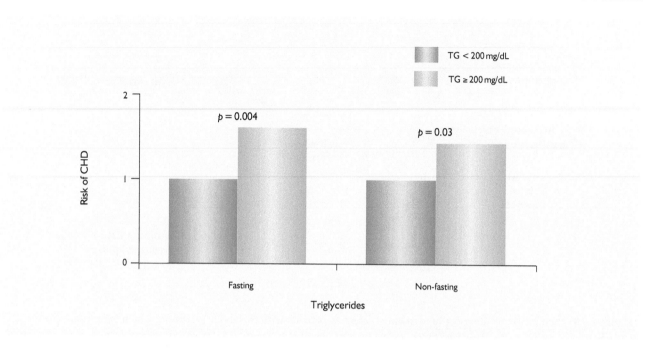

Figure 5.17 Data from the MR FIT study showing the adjusted risk of a fatal or non-fatal CHD event in relation to a fasting or non-fasting triglyceride (TG) level of ≥ 200 mg/dL. Compared with a TG of < 200 mg/dL, a TG of ≥ 200 mg/dL was associated with a 46–64% increased risk, independent of other risk factors including lipid parameters. From reference 22, with permission

the high triglyceride/low HDL cholesterol lipid profile commonly observed in insulin resistant subjects.

Hypertriglyceridemia is a strong predictor of coronary heart disease. Prospective studies such as MR FIT study show that the adjusted risk of a fatal or non-fatal CHD event is greater in subjects with a triglyceride (TG) level of ≥ 200 mg/dL (Figure 5.17)[22]. This is irrespective of whether the subjects were in a fasting or non fasting state. The Whitehall II study showed that the potential relevance of combining TG and cholesterol in risk prediction (Figure 5.18)[23]. There is also an inverse relationship between serum levels of HDL cholesterol and triglycerides, with low serum HDL cholesterol levels representing an independent risk factor for cardiovascular disease and the so-called 'atherogenic lipid triad' consists of high serum triglyceride levels, low serum HDL cholesterol levels, and a preponderance of small, dense, low-density lipoprotein (LDL) cholesterol particles. Small, dense, LDL cholesterol particles are also highly atherogenic as they are more likely to form oxidized LDL and are less readily cleared, hence LDL particle size is a powerful predictor of cardiovascular risk (Figure 5.19). Epidemiological studies show a strong linear relationship between the number of small dense LDL particles are subsequent risk of adverse clinical events (Figure 5.19)[24] Therefore, measurement of LDL cholesterol does not give the most accurate measurement of the number of atherogenic particles in subjects with the metabolic syndrome. For this reason some have advocated the use of non-HDL cholesterol in risk stratification or the measurement of apolipoprotein B which measures the total number of atherogenic particles present (LDL, VLDL and inter-mediate-density lipoprotein (IDL)) (Figure 5.20 and 5.21)[25,26]. In the AMORIS study there was a linear relationship with respect to apoB levels and risk of fatal MI[25]. In the Women's Health Study the risk of cardiovascular events increased with increasing quintiles of non-HDL cholesterol, or quintiles of apolipoprotein B[26].

HYPERTENSION

Elevated blood pressure has been recognized as a risk factor for cardiovascular disease for several decades and the definition of what constitutes hypertension

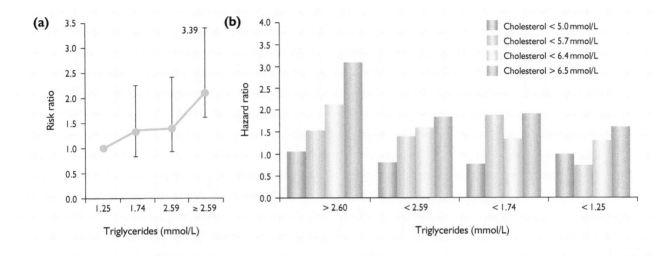

Figure 5.18 Data from the Whitehall II study showing the isolated and combined predictive value of incremental non-fasting triglyceride (TG) levels and subsequent risk of CHD events. (a) Univariate relative risk of CHD events in quartiles of TG. (b) Stratification of proportion of CHD events by quartiles of TG and cholesterol. From reference 23, with permission

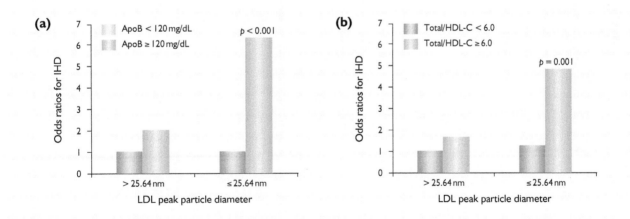

Figure 5.19 Data from the Quebec Heart Study showing the odds ratios for ischemic heart disease (IHD) and probability levels according to apolipoprotein (apo) B levels (a), the total/HDL cholesterol ratio (b), and LDL peak particle diameter (PPD). The median of the distribution of apoB (120 mg/dL) and the total/HDL-C ratio (6.0) were used to classify men as having low or elevated levels for these variables. For the present analysis, men with small LDL particles (LDL-PPD ≤ 25.64 nm) were compared with those having intermediate and large LDL particles (LDL-PPD > 25.64 nm). Individuals with small LDL particles in the absence of elevated apoB concentrations (apoB levels < 120 mg/dL, the median value of the distribution) were not at increased risk for IHD compared with men with larger LDL particles and with relatively low apoB levels. Elevated apoB concentrations among individuals with large LDL particles resulted in a two-fold increase in IHD risk, which did not reach statistical significance. Among these four groups, individuals having both elevated apoB levels and small LDL particles showed the greatest increase in IHD risk (OR 6.2; 95% CI 2.2–17.4; $p < 0.001$). A similar association was observed between LDL-PPD and the total/HDL cholesterol ratio, because only men with small LDL particles and with an elevated total/HDL cholesterol ratio were at greater risk of IHD (OR 4.9; 95% CI 1.9–12.7) compared with men having both large LDL particles and a ratio < 6. From reference 24, with permission

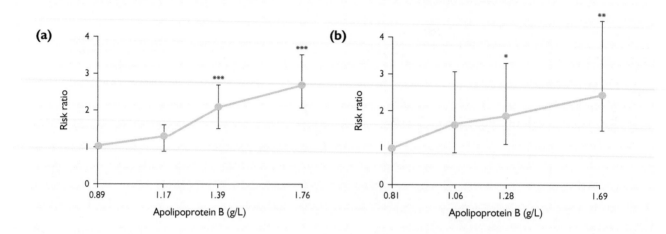

Figure 5.20 Data from the AMORIS study showing the age-adjusted risk of fatal myocardial infarction with respect to apoB levels (log transformed) for men (a) and women (b). With increasing apoB levels the risk of fatal MI increases. From reference 25, with permission. $^{*}p < 0.05$; $^{**}p < 0.001$; $^{***}p < 0.0001$

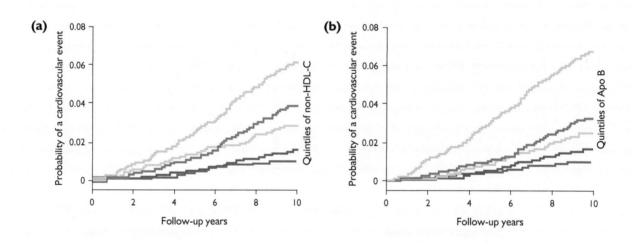

Figure 5.21 Data from the Women's Health Study showing the probability of a cardiovascular event across increasing quintiles of non-HDL cholesterol (a) or quintiles of apolipoprotein B (b). Similar information was provided by using non-HDL-C as apoB. From reference 26, with permission

has been progressively lowered. Hypertension is an important constituent of the metabolic syndrome and is well established as an important risk factor for cardiovascular disease. Several types of hypertension have defined causes, such as renovascular hypertension (Figure 2.22)[7] or Berger's disease (Figure 5.23)[7], but the exact nature of the genesis of hypertension in

the metabolic syndrome is unclear. A possible link is that among subjects with insulin resistance, hyperglycemia leads to glycation and cross-linking of collagen, resulting in reduced elasticity and increased arterial stiffness. In animal studies breaking these cross-links results in a restoration of elasticity, further supporting the potential role of glycation of collagen

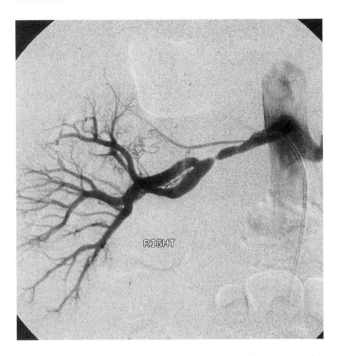

Figure 5.22 Digital subtraction angiogram showing a tight renal artery stenosis due to localized fibromuscular dyplasia in a 27-year-old nurse who had hypertension. Longer stenotic segments often present with a 'string-of-beads' appearance. From reference 7, with permission

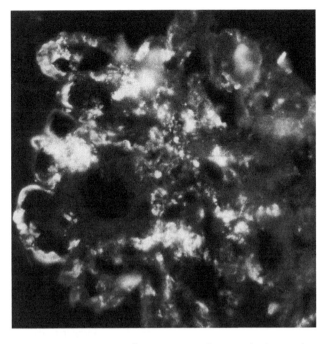

Figure 5.23 Immunoflourescence of a renal glomerulus showing granular deposits of IgA immune complex (yellow-green) mainly in the mesangium, typical of IgA nephropathy (Berger's disease). Patients with IgA nephropathy often present with hypertension, and are usually positive on urine stick tests for blood and protein. From reference 7, with permission

in the etiology of hypertension among subjects with the metabolic syndrome.

In a recent individual participant meta-analysis the age-specific relationship between blood pressure and cause-specific mortality was assessed in 1 million adults with no previous vascular disease recorded at baseline in 61 prospective observational studies (Figure 5.24)[27]. During 12.7 million person years at risk, there were 56 000 vascular deaths at ages 40–89 years. Within each decade of age at death, the proportional difference in the risk of vascular death associated with a given absolute difference in usual blood pressure was about the same down to 115 mmHg systolic and 75 mmHg diastolic blood pressure. At ages 40–69 years, each difference of 20 mmHg systolic blood pressure (or, approximately equivalently, 10 mmHg diastolic blood pressure) was associated with more than a two-fold difference in the stroke death rate, and with two-fold differences in the death rates from ischemic heart disease and from other vascular causes. All of these proportional differences in vascular mortality are about half as extreme at ages

80–89 years as at ages 40–49 years, but the annual absolute difference in risk was greater in old age. The age-specific associations were similar for men and women, and for cerebral hemorrhage or ischemia. For predicting vascular mortality from a single blood pressure, the average of systolic and diastolic blood pressure was slightly more informative than either alone, and pulse pressure was much less informative.

There are important consequences of hypertension which could contribute to cardiovascular risk (Figure 5.25) Elevated blood pressure results in increased vasoreactivity and endothelial dysfunction and increased oxidative stress. These changes contribute to the endothelial dysfunction and inflammation. Additionally raised blood pressure increases hydrostatic pressure thus increasing the deposition of atherogenic particles in the vessel wall. Increased after-load contributes to the deterioration in renal function and also left ventricular diastolic dysfunction and later systolic dysfunction resulting in heart failure. Although hypertension is a component of the metabolic syndrome, cardiovascular risk is increased

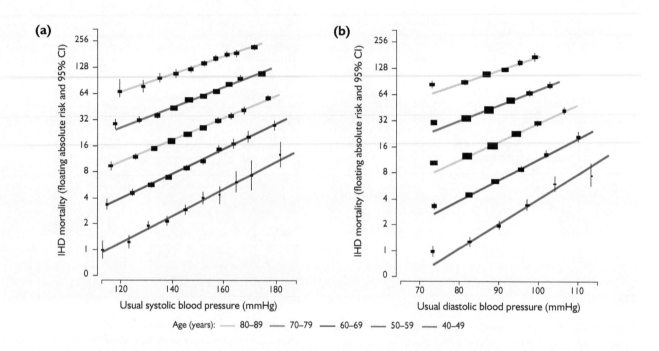

Figure 5.24 Data from the prospective studies collaboration showing the linear relationship between systolic (a) and diastolic (b) blood pressure and mortality from ischemic heart disease (IHD) across decades of age. The data show the relationship between blood pressure and risk of events is equal across each decade of age. However, as aging increases risk per se, the risk of any given blood pressure increases with age. From reference 27, with permission

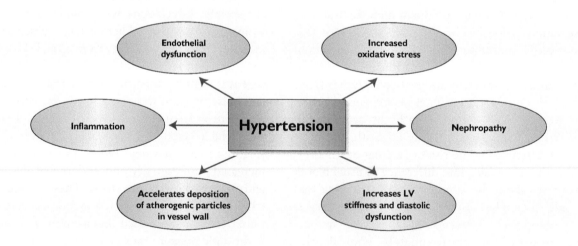

Figure 5.25 Schematic showing the pathological consequences of hypertension. Elevated blood pressure results in increased vasoreactivity and endothelial dysfunction. Increased oxidative stress may further contribute to the endothelial dysfunction and inflammation. Increased hydrostatic pressure increases the deposition of atherogenic particles in the vessel wall. Increased afterload contributes to the deterioration in renal function which may further exacerbate hypertension. Increased afterload results in increased left ventricular (LV) stiffness and diastolic dysfunction, and later systolic dysfunction

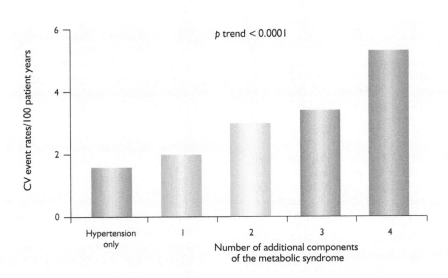

Figure 5.26 Data showing the prognostic additive effect of the number of additional components of the metabolic syndrome and risk of cardiovascular events among subjects with hypertension. Over 10 years the risk of cardiovascular events increased with each additional component of the metabolic syndrome (increased BMI, triglycerides, glucose, or low HDL), showing the synergistic effect of additional metabolic risk factors. From reference 28, with permission

with each additional component of the syndrome (Figure 5.26)[28].

REFERENCES

1. Kannel WB, McGee DL. Diabetes and cardiovascular disease. The Framingham study. JAMA 1979; 241: 2035–8

2. Standl E, Balletshofer B, Dahl B, et al. Predictors of 10year macrovascular and overall mortality in patients with NIDDM: the Munich General Practitioner Project. Diabetologia 1996; 39: 1540–5

3. Khaw KT, Wareham N, Luben R, et al. Glycated haemoglobin, diabetes, and mortality in men in Norfolk cohort of European Prospective Investigation of Cancer and Nutrition (EPIC-Norfolk). Br Med J 2001; 322: 15

4. Nathan DM, Cleary PA, Blacklund JY, et al.; Diabetes Control and Complications Trial/Epidemiology of Diabetes Interventions and Complications (DCCT/EDIC) Study Research Group. Intensive diabetes treatment and cardiovascular disease in patients with type 1 diabetes. N Engl J Med 2005; 353: 2643–53

5. Dormandy JA, Charbonnel B, Eckland DJ, et al. Secondary prevention of macrovascular events in patients with type 2 diabetes in the PROactive Study (PROspective pioglitAzone Clinical Trial In macroVascular Events): a randomised controlled trial. Lancet 2005; 366: 1279–89

6. Kilhovd BK, Juutilainen A, Lehto S, et al. High serum levels of advanced glycation end products predict increased coronary heart disease mortality in nondiabetic women but not in nondiabetic men: a population-based 18-year follow-up study. Arterioscler Thromb Vasc Biol 2005; 25: 815–20

7. Semple PF, Lindop GBM. An Atlas of Hypertension. Carnforth, UK: Parthenon Publishing, 1992

8. Stary HC. Atlas of Atherosclerosis: Progression and Regression, 2nd edn. Lancaster, UK: Parthenon Publishing, 2003: 104

9. Brewer HB Jr. Increasing HDL cholesterol levels. N Engl J Med 2004; 350: 1491–4

10. Gordon DJ, Probstfield JL, Garrison RJ, et al. High-density lipoprotein cholesterol and cardiovascular disease. Four prospective American studies. Circulation 1989; 79: 8–15

11. Gordon T, Castelli WP, Hjortland MC, et al. High density lipoprotein as a protective factor against coronary heart disease. The Framingham Study. Am J Med 1977; 62: 707–14

12. Multiple risk factor intervention trial. Risk factor changes and mortality results. Multiple Risk Factor Intervention Trial Research Group. JAMA 1982; 248: 1465–77

13. Assmann G, Schulte H, von Eckardstein A, Huang Y. High-density lipoprotein cholesterol as a predictor of coronary heart disease risk. The PROCAM experience and pathophysiological implications for reverse cholesterol transport. Atherosclerosis 1996; 124 (Suppl): S11–20

14. Jacobs DR Jr, Mebane IL, Bangdiwala SI, et al. High density lipoprotein cholesterol as a predictor of cardiovascular disease mortality in men and women: the follow-up study of the Lipid Research Clinics Prevalence Study. Am J Epidemiol 1990; 131: 32–47

15. Gordon DJ, Knoke J, Probstfield JL, et al. High-density lipoprotein cholesterol and coronary heart disease in hypercholesterolemic men: the Lipid Research Clinics Coronary Primary Prevention Trial. Circulation 1986; 74: 1217–25

16. Burchfiel CM, Laws A, Benfante R, et al. Combined effects of HDL cholesterol, triglyceride, and total cholesterol concentrations on 18-year risk of atherosclerotic disease. Circulation 1995; 92: 1430–6

17. Sacks FM, Tonkin AM, Craven T, et al. Coronary heart disease in patients with low LDL-cholesterol: benefit of pravastatin in diabetics and enhanced role for HDL-cholesterol and triglycerides as risk factors. Circulation 2002; 105: 1424–8

18. Grundy SM, Cleeman JI, Merz CN, et al. Implications of recent clinical trials for the National Cholesterol Education Program Adult Treatment Panel III guidelines. Circulation 2004; 110: 227–39

19. Chapman MJ, Assmann G, Fruchart JC, et al. Raising high-density lipoprotein cholesterol with reduction of cardiovascular risk: the role of nicotinic acid: a position paper developed by the European Consensus Panel on HDL-C. Curr Med Res Opin 2004; 20: 1253–68

20. Birjmohun RS, Hutten BA, Kastelein JJ, Stroes ES. Efficacy and safety of high-density lipoprotein cholesterol-increasing compounds: a meta-analysis of randomized controlled trials. J Am Coll Cardiol 2005; 45: 185–97

21. Taylor AJ, Sullenberger LE, Lee HJ, et al. Arterial Biology for the Investigation of the Treatment Effects of Reducing Cholesterol (ARBITER) 2: a double-blind, placebo-controlled study of extended-release niacin on atherosclerosis progression in secondary prevention patients treated with statins. Circulation 2004; 110: 3512–17

22. Eberly LE, Stamler J, Neaton JD. Relation of triglyceride levels, fasting and nonfasting, to fatal and nonfatal coronary heart disease. Arch Intern Med 2003; 163: 1077–83

23. Talmud PJ, Hawe E, Miller GJ, Humphries SE. Nonfasting apolipoprotein B and triglyceride levels as a useful predictor of coronary heart disease risk in middle-aged UK men. Arterioscler Thromb Vasc Biol 2002; 22: 1918–23

24. Lamarche BA, Tchernof S, Moorjani B, et al. Small, dense low-density lipoprotein particles as a predictor of the risk of ischemic heart disease in men: prospective results from the Quebec cardiovascular study. Circulation 1997; 95: 69–75

25. Walldius GI, Jungner I, Holme AH, et al. High apolipoprotein B, low apolipoprotein A-I, and improvement in the prediction of fatal myocardial infarction (AMORIS study): a prospective study. Lancet 2001; 358: 2026–33

26. Ridker PM, et al. Non-HDL-choelsterol, apolipoproteins A-I and B-100, standard lipid measures, lipid ratios, and CRP as risk for cardiovascular disease in women. JAMA 2005; 294: 326–33

27. Lewington S, Clarke R, Qizilbash N, et al. Age-specific relevance of usual blood pressure to vascular mortality: a meta-analysis of individual data for one million adults in 61 prospective studies. Lancet 2002; 360: 1903–13

28. Schillaci GM, Pirro G, Vaudo F, et al. Prognostic value of the metabolic syndrome in essential hypertension. J Am Coll Cardiol 2004; 43: 1817–22

6   Non-traditional risk factors of cardiometabolic risk

INFLAMMATION AND CARDIOVASCULAR RISK

Inflammation is an intrinsic part of the pathogenesis of atherosclerosis and cardiovascular disease (CVD)[1]. Accumulation of inflammatory cells in the vessel wall and predominantly in so-called vulnerable plaques suggests that the most vulnerable sites in the vessel wall have the most intense inflammatory activity[2,3]. Inflammatory cells whether in the vessel wall or the circulation produce a number of inflammatory proteins called cytokines which are central to the proinflammatory response of the vessel wall and the systemic acute phase response. Inflammatory cytokines such as interleukin-1 (IL-1) and interleukin-6 (IL-6) stimulate the production of C-reactive protein (CRP) predominantly by the liver, but also by endothelial and smooth muscle cells in the vessel wall (Figure 6.1).

INTERLEUKIN-6

Interleukin (IL)-6 is a pluripotent cytokine with a broad range of humoral and cellular immune effects relating to inflammation, host defense, and tissue injury (Figure 6.2). It is produced in response to several factors, including infection; other cytokines, such as IL-1, interferon-γ, and tumor necrosis factor; and is the central mediator of the acute-phase response and the primary determinant of hepatic production of CRP. Inflammatory cells as well as endothelial and smooth muscle cells produce IL-6. In apparently healthy individuals levels of IL-6 increase with an increase in the number of traditional risk factors present[4]. In addition, several epidemiological studies have demonstrated a positive correlation between increasing IL-6 and cardiovascular events (Figure 6.3)[4,5].

C-REACTIVE PROTEIN

Several studies have shown that there is a significant relationship between individual components of the metabolic syndrome and CRP. The exact relationship varies from component to component (Figure 6.4), but broadly there is a positive relationship with blood pressure, glucose, insulin resistance, obesity, and triglycerides, and a negative relationship with HDL. That CRP levels correspond with individual components of the metabolic syndrome is consistent with the hypothesized role of inflammation in several processes critical to the development of atherothrombosis. Furthermore, several cross-sectional studies have demonstrated that there is a positive relationship between the number of components of the metabolic syndrome and CRP[6,7] (Figure 6.5). Among healthy populations such as the Women's Health Study the average CRP levels are higher among subjects with the metabolic syndrome (average range 3.01–5.75 mg/L) compared with those without (average range 0.68–1.93 mg/L). Thus, some researchers have suggested that CRP may be a useful 'global barometer' of cardiovascular risk factor burden[6].

It has now emerged that CRP rather than being an innocent bystander and a mere marker of systemic inflammation, may also, in part, directly have adverse

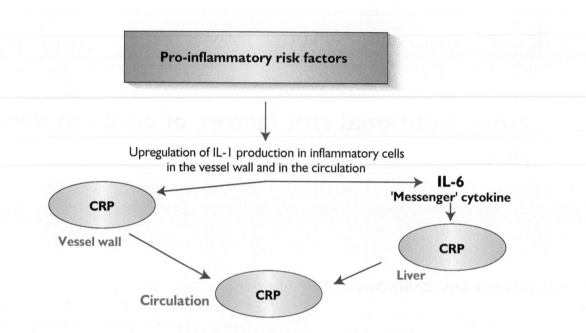

Figure 6.1 Schematic demonstrating the cytokine 'cascade' leading to the production of CRP. The presence of inflammatory risk factors results in the increased production of the 'apical' proinflammatory cytokine interleukin (IL)-1 by various inflammatory cells. IL-1 in turn drives the increased production of a second downstream 'messenger' cytokine IL-6, which is the principal determinant of CRP production mostly by the liver, and to a lesser degree by the vessel wall

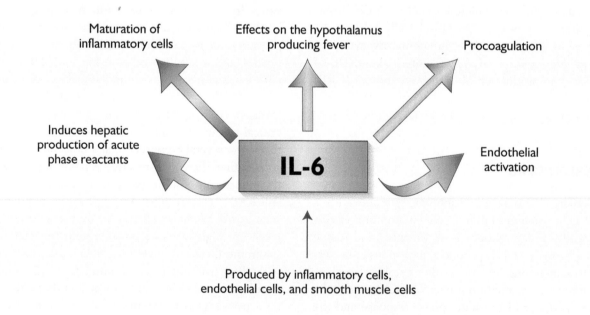

Figure 6.2 Schematic of the multiple biological effects of IL-6. IL-6 plays an important role in driving the inflammatory response by effects on inflammatory cells and the production of acute phase reactants and fever. It also has effects on coagulation and endothelial activation

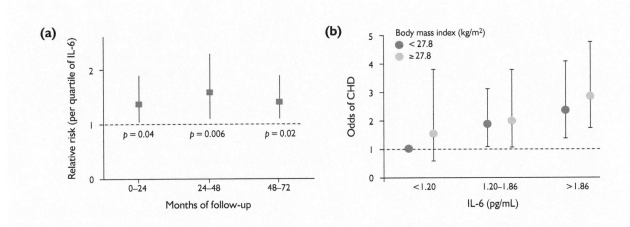

Figure 6.3 Data showing the risk of incident myocardial infarction in apparently healthy men, per increasing quartile of IL-6 (a) and the odds of CHD in postmenopausal women (b). With increasing IL-6 levels the risk of events increases. From references 4 and 5, with permission

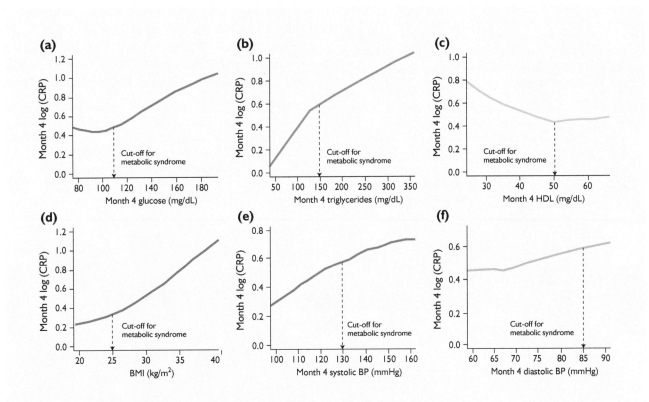

Figure 6.4 Relationship between individual components of the metabolic syndrome (x axis) and CRP (y axis) from the PROVE IT-TIMI 22 trial. In this analysis Ray *et al.* demonstrated that for many of the components of the metabolic syndrome such as glucose, diastolic BP, and HDL there were thresholds below or above which CRP remained fairly constant despite the change in the risk factor. These thresholds may be useful targets in future for reducing inflammation. In contrast, an almost linear relationship was observed between systolic blood pressure, triglycerides, and BMI. From reference 6, with permission

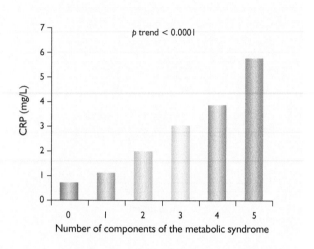

Figure 6.5 Relationship between the number of components of the metabolic syndrome and CRP in 14 719 apparently healthy women, in the Women's Health Study (values shown are median levels). As the number of components increase, so does CRP with an average increase of approximately 1 mg/L for each additional component of the metabolic syndrome. For women without any component of the syndrome CRP levels were 0.68 mg/L and for those with every component the corresponding value was 5.75 mg/L. From reference 8, with permission

pathological effects. This suggests that CRP is an important 'player' as well as a marker of cardiovascular risk (Figure 6.6). Its actions include adverse biological effects on the vessel wall and on coagulation[9]. In response to CRP, the vessel wall produces proteins called adhesion molecules, which are able to bind circulating inflammatory cells. These inflammatory cells migrate into the vessel wall and release proteolytic enzymes and inflammatory proteins which lead to plaque rupture. Furthermore, CRP stimulates the release of tissue factor from inflammatory cells which can lead to clot formation.

More than 20 prospective studies have demonstrated a relationship between elevated CRP and risk of future cardiovascular disease. Using cut-offs of < 1, 1–3, and > 3 there is a linear relationship between increasing CRP levels and CVD risk. For instance, the Physicians' Health Study (PHS)[10], the Women's Health Study (WHS)[11], Monitoring of Trends and Determinants of Cardiovascular disease (MONICA) study[12] and the Atherosclerosis Risk in Communities study (ARIC)[13] demonstrated that a CRP > 3 mg/L carried a nearly 2-fold excess risk of cardiovascular events compared with a CRP level < 1 mg/L, which was independent of other risk factors (Figure 6.7).

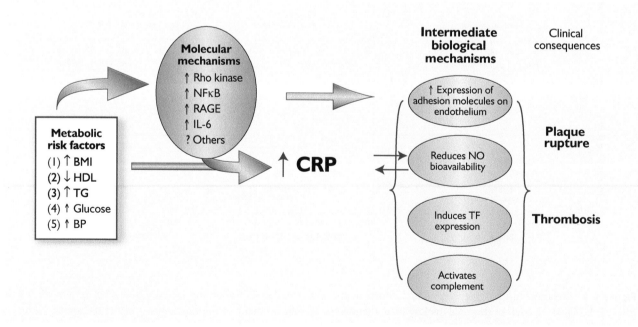

Figure 6.6 Schematic demonstrating the proinflammatory effects of CRP. NFκB, nuclear factor kappa B; RAGE, receptor for advanced glycation end products; TF, tissue factor

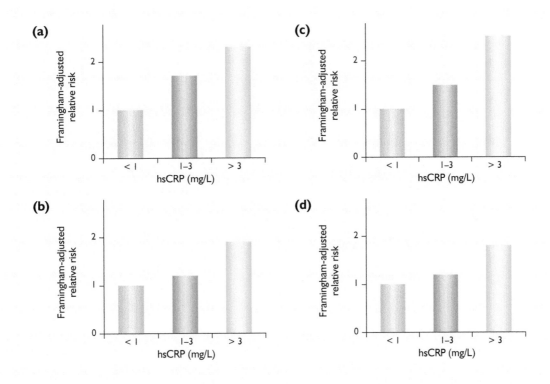

Figure 6.7 The relationship between low-grade systemic inflammation and risk of coronary events in the PHS (a), WHS (b), MONICA (c) and ARIC (d) studies. After adjustment for Framingham risk factors there is an incremental relative risk with increasing high-sensitivity (hs)CRP levels. From reference 14, with permission

Significantly, several studies have demonstrated that CRP adds prognostic information on cardiovascular risk above and beyond that available using the Framingham risk score alone. The Pravastatin Inflammation/CRP Evaluation (PRINCE) database has provided evidence that CRP picks up risk information that cannot be gleaned from the individual Framingham covariates[15,16]. Since nearly two-thirds of first coronary events occur in individuals who would otherwise be considered at low or moderate risk based on the Framingham risk calculation, this suggests that additional markers or factors causal in CVD await discovery. In groups of patients at moderate to low risk who would otherwise not be identified, CRP levels provide further risk stratification in prospective studies.

Several cardiovascular risk factors increase the atherogenic potential of other risk factors when present in combination. For example, high glucose levels modify LDL cholesterol and make LDL cholesterol more atherogenic. Data from the PROVE-IT TIMI 22 trial demonstrate that in addition to correlating with several risk factors, CRP levels 'detect' the interaction between risk factors such as LDL cholesterol and glucose, thus providing additional information regarding synergistic effects of combinations of risk factors (Figure 6.8).

Data from the WHS show that at every level of the Framingham risk score CRP levels provide additional independent prognostic information, beyond traditional risk factors. Whether the Framingham risk estimate is < 1% or 10–20%, a CRP > 3 mg/L carries approximately a 2-fold excess risk of CHD vs. a CRP < 1 mg/L (Figure 6.9).

Among patients at low (Framingham 10-year risk of < 10%) or at intermediate risk (Framingham 10-year risk of 10–20%) more extreme high-sensitivity (hs)CRP levels of > 10 mg/L carry a nearly 4.5-fold excess risk compared with those with a CRP

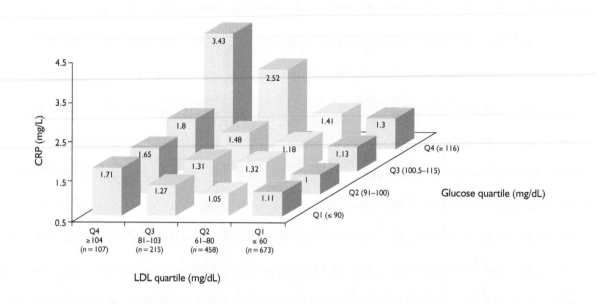

Figure 6.8 Data from the PROVE-IT TIMI 22 trial showing that in addition to correlating with several risk factors, CRP levels 'detect' the interaction between risk factors such as LDL cholesterol and glucose, thus providing additional information regarding synergistic effects of combinations of risk factors. A statistically significant interaction ($p = 0.034$) was observed between increasing LDL and glucose levels. From reference 6, with permission

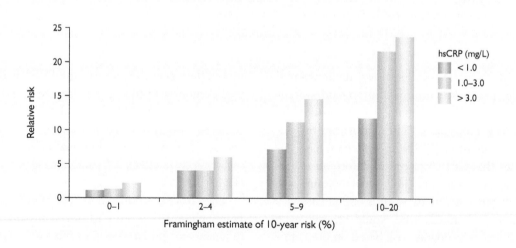

Figure 6.9 Data from the WHS showing that at every level of the Framingham risk score CRP levels provide additional independent prognostic information, beyond traditional risk factors. From reference 17, with permission

< 0.5 mg/L (Figure 6.10). Data from the Women's Health Study further demonstrate the important relationship between inflammation and cardiovascular risk.

Among patients with the metabolic syndrome, the Women's Health Study demonstrated that at all levels of severity of the metabolic syndrome, CRP added important and independent prognostic information in

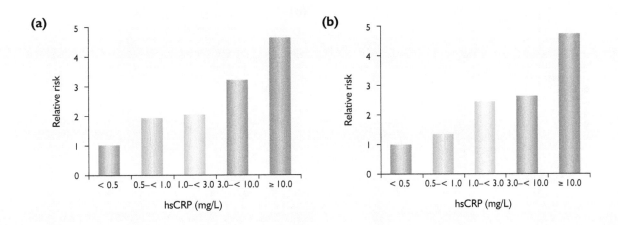

Figure 6.10 Predictive value of high-sensitivity (hs)CRP in calculating the relative risks of future cardiovascular events in patients at low (Framingham 10-year risk < 10%) (a) and intermediate risk (Framingham 10-year risk 10–20%) (b). From reference 17, with permission

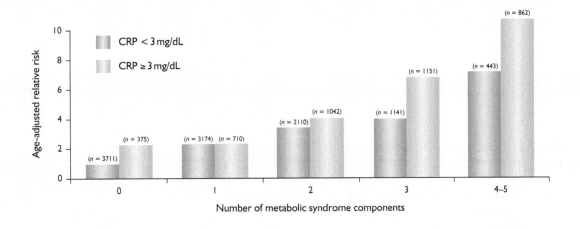

Figure 6.11 Data from the Women's Health Study demonstrating that a CRP > 3 mg/L provides further prognostic information beyond that provided by the components of the metabolic syndrome. The impact of CRP > 3 mg/L and cardiovascular risk was most apparent among those with three or more components of the metabolic syndrome. From reference 8, with permission

terms of future cardiovascular risk. This additive effect was present in all study groups evaluated including those with LDL cholesterol above and below 130 mg/dL and was applicable to the different methods used to define the metabolic syndrome. The prog-nostic benefit of CRP also added to the information obtained from assessing whether the metabolic syndrome was present or absent (Figure 6.11). Similar data were observed in the West of Scotland Pravastatin Study (WOSCOPS) which assessed only male patients

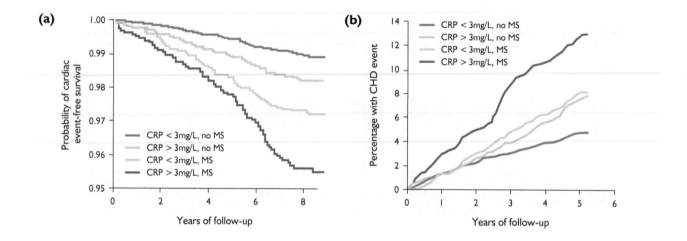

Figure 6.12 Among both women (Women's Health Study) (a) and men (WOSCOPS) (b) a CRP > 3 mg/L identifies groups of patients at high and low risk. Among patients without the metabolic syndrome (MS), a CRP < 3 mg/L identifies the lowest risk group. Among subjects with the metabolic syndrome a CRP > 3 mg/L further identifies a group at high risk of cardiac events, with subjects having the metabolic syndrome and a high CRP being at greatest risk. Those subjects without the metabolic syndrome and a high CRP or with the metabolic syndrome and a low CRP were at intermediate risk. From references 8 and 18, with permission

(Figure 6.12). The metabolic syndrome is believed to antecede the development of diabetes. In the WOSCOPS study the presence of CRP ≥ 3 mg/L was a better predictor of new-onset diabetes than the metabolic syndrome alone.

PLASMINOGEN-ACTIVATOR INHIBITOR TYPE 1

In health there is an intrinsic balance between thrombus formation and fibrinolysis. Tissue plasminogen activator (t-PA) is the human body's endogenous fibrinolytic which is produced by the endothelium. Plasminogen-activator inhibitor (PAI) is the natural inhibitor of t-PA which is also produced by the vessel wall. Normally the net balance between t-PA and PAI-1 favors fibrinolysis. However, in response to an inflammatory stimulus, such as IL-1 or CRP, the expression and release of PAI-1 is increased. At the same time the expression and release of t-PA falls, resulting in 'hypofibrinolysis.' Histological staining of vulnerable coronary athrosclerotic plaques obtained by atherectomy shows increased expression of tissue factor (favoring thrombosis) and increased expression

of PAI-1, suggesting that an imbalance between coagulation and fibrinolysis contributes to the pathogenesis of acute coronary events.

The main coagulation reactions are divided into the intrinsic and extrinsic systems (Figure 6.13). Activation of factor XII on contact with a negatively charged surface initiates the intrinsic coagulation system. (The activated form of a factor is indicated by 'a'.) The extrinsic coagulation system induces the formation of a complex composed of factor VII and tissue factor, which is released after tissue injury. Intrinsic and extrinsic activation of the coagulation cascade leads to the generation of thrombin, the activation of fibrinogen, the release of fibrinopeptides, the formation of soluble fibrin, and, finally, the formation of factor XIII-mediated, cross-linked, insoluble fibrin. The main fibrinolytic reactions involve the inhibition of fibrinolysis by PAI-1 and α_2-antiplasmin. Fibrinolysis is initiated by t-PA, urinary-type plasminogen activator (u-PA), and plasmin. Plasmin bound to the surface of fibrin initiates the lysis of insoluble, cross-linked fibrin, with the subsequent generation of fibrin-degradation products. Plasmin bound to the surface of fibrin is better protected from inhibition by α_2-antiplasmin than is plasmin generated in the fluid phase[16].

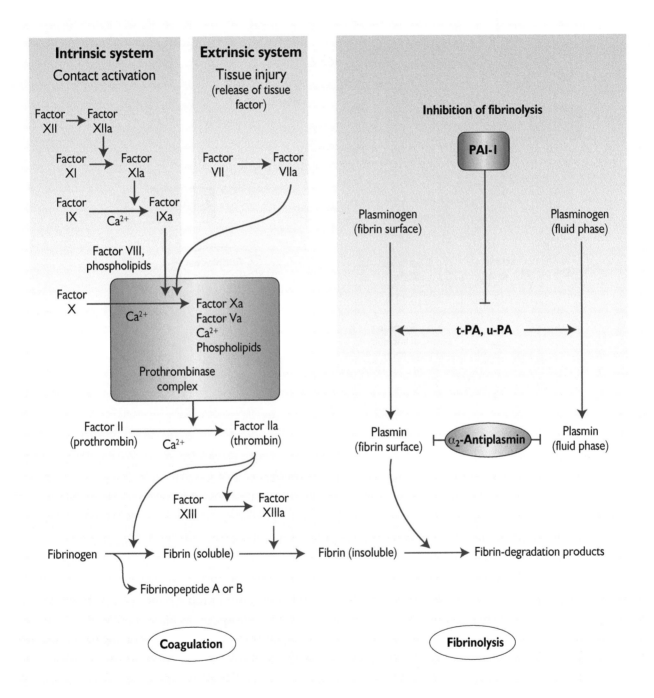

Figure 6.13 The main coagulation reactions are divided into the intrinsic and extrinsic systems. Activation of factor XII on contact with a negatively charged surface initiates the intrinsic coagulation system. (The activated form of the factor is indicated by 'a'.) The extrinsic coagulation system induces the formation of a complex composed of factor VII and tissue factor, which is released after tissue injury. Intrinsic and extrinsic activation of the coagulation cascade leads to the generation of thrombin, the activation of fibrinogen, the release of fibrinopeptides, the formation of soluble fibrin, and, finally, the formation of factor XIII-mediated, cross-linked, insoluble fibrin. The main fibrinolytic reactions involve the inhibition of fibrinolysis by plasminogen-activator inhibitor type 1 (PAI-1) and α_2-antiplasmin. Fibrinolysis is initiated by tissue plasminogen activator (t-PA), urinary-type plasminogen activator (u-PA), and plasmin. Plasmin bound to the surface of fibrin initiates the lysis of insoluble, cross-linked fibrin, with the subsequent generation of fibrin-degradation products. Plasmin bound to the surface of fibrin is better protected from inhibition by α_2-antiplasmin than is plasmin generated in the fluid phase. From reference 16, with permission

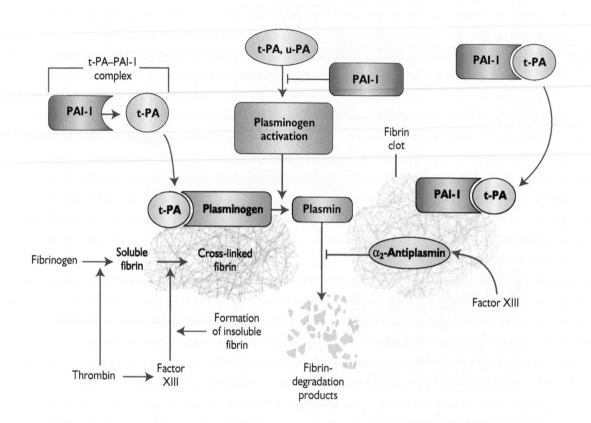

Figure 6.14 Schematic of activation and inhibition of the fibrinolytic pathway. Tissue plasminogen activator (t-PA) circulates in plasma as a complex with plasminogen-activator inhibitor type 1 (PAI-1) in a 1 : 1 ratio. The fibrin clot provides the surface on which the reactions occur. Plasminogen is activated by t-PA or urinary-type plasminogen activator (u-PA). Plasminogen, t-PA, and fibrin form a ternary complex that promotes the formation of plasmin and the subsequent lysis of cross-linked fibrin into low-molecular-weight fragments (fibrin-degradation products). PAI-1 also binds to fibrin and, when bound, retains its inhibitory activity against t-PA. α_2-Antiplasmin is cross-linked to fibrin by factor XIII. From reference 16, with permission

Epidemiological evidence suggests that circulating PAI-1 levels are elevated in patients with coronary heart disease and may play an important role in the development of atherothrombosis. Many clinical studies have indicated that the metabolic syndrome is associated with elevated plasma PAI-1 levels. PAI-1 is also positively correlated with insulin, blood pressure, and triglyceride levels, and negatively to HDL cholesterol[19–21]. Central obesity which is a characteristic of the metabolic syndrome may be particularly relevant to the increased levels of PAI-1. Although PAI-1 is predominantly of endothelial origin the production of PAI-1 by adipose tissue, in particular by tissue from the omentum, has also been demonstrated and could be an important contributor to the elevated plasma

PAI-1 levels observed in metabolic syndrome patients[22]. Prospective cohort studies of patients with previous myocardial infarction or angina pectoris have underlined the association between increased plasma PAI-1 levels and the risk of recurrent coronary events, but the predictive capacity of PAI-1 is reduced after adjustment for markers of insulin resistance[23]. Taken together these results support the notion that PAI-1 can be a link between obesity, insulin resistance, and cardiovascular disease.

In the PRIME study of nearly 10 500 subjects, PAI-1 activity increased with body mass index, waist-to-hip ratio, triglycerides, alcohol intake, and smoking, and decreased with leisure physical activity. PAI-1 level was higher in diabetic subjects than in subjects

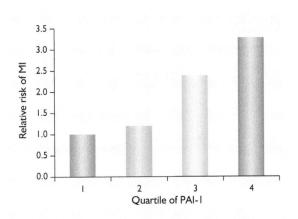

Figure 6.15 The data shown demonstrates that among patients with PAI-1 levels in quartile 4 there is an approximately three-fold excess risk compared with those in the lowest quartile, $p < 0.0001$. This risk was attenuated after adjustment for traditional risk factors. From reference 25, with permission

without diabetes. Cardiovascular risk factors explained 26% of the total variance in PAI-1. The odds ratio for cardiovascular disease associated with a rise of one standard deviation in PAI-1 was 1.38 (95% CI 1.27–1.49, $p < 0.001$). After adjustment for cardiovascular risk factors, this association was attenuated but remained highly significant. Similarly data from the prospective Northwick Park Heart Study also demonstrated a strong, long-term relationship between a low level of plasma fibrinolytic activity at enrollment and the subsequent incidence of coronary artery disease in young men, suggesting that low fibrinolytic activity precedes heart disease[24]. In prospective studies of healthy subjects at risk of myocardial infarction a linear relationship between increasing PAI-1 and risk of first myocardial infarction has been observed (Figure 6.15).

ENDOTHELIAL DYSFUNCTION

Over the past two decades, it has become evident that the endothelium is more than an inert, single-cell lining covering the internal surface of blood vessels. Normally, the endothelium actively decreases vascular tone by producing nitric oxide, maintains vascular permeability within narrow bounds, inhibits platelet adhesion and aggregation, limits activation of the coagulation system, and stimulates fibrinolysis. Endothelial dysfunction can be considered present when its functions, either in the basal state or after stimulation, are altered in a way that is inappropriate to the preservation of organ function. Endothelial dysfunction has been associated to many cardiovascular risk factors including diabetes, hypertension, and hypercholesterolemia. In addition, endothelial dysfunction may play a crucial role in the development and progression of atherosclerosis.

The normal healthy endothelium produces nitric oxide (NO) and very little endothelin-1 stimulating vasodilatation. There is very little expression of adhesion molecules, such as E-selectin or ICAM, which reduces platelet and inflammatory cell adhesion to the vessel wall. Production of thrombomodulin (the intrinsic natural anticoagulant) on the vessel wall binds thrombin which then activates protein C (which forms the body's natural anticoagulant cascade). In subjects with endothelial dysfunction nitric oxide production is reduced and endothelin production increased favoring vasoconstriction, adhesion molecules are expressed which bind inflammatory cells, and tissue factor is expressed with very little thrombomodulin favoring thrombus formation (Figure 6.16).

Studies have investigated which components of the metabolic syndrome are closely linked with endothelial dysfunction as assessed by changes in coronary flow in response to an agonist (Figure 6.17)[26]. Specifically waist circumference, systolic blood pressure, and insulin resistance were significantly negatively correlated with coronary vasodilatation. This suggests the greater the extent of obesity, the higher the blood pressure and the greater the extent of insulin resistance the worse the degree of endothelial dysfunction[26].

Halcox *et al.* studied the relationship between endothelium-dependent coronary vascular function and acute cardiovascular events in subjects with angiographically normal coronary arteries. Subjects with the greatest vasodilator reserve had the lowest incidence of acute cardiovascular events (Figure 6.18)[27]. Similar findings have been observed in subjects with mild angiographic coronary disease[28].

The integrity of the vessel wall depends upon the ability of the body to repair the damaged endothelium. Central to this are the bone marrow-derived

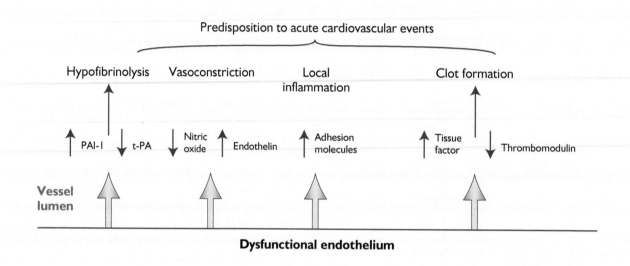

Figure 6.16 Schematic of dysfunctional endothelium. PAI-1, plasminogen-activator inhibitor type 1; t-PA, tissue plasminogen activator

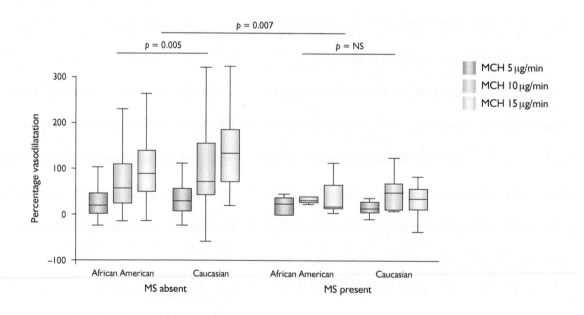

Figure 6.17 Under normal conditions there is an increasing vasodilator response to increasing doses of the agonist metacholine (MCH) in Caucasians and African Americans. This relationship is significantly attenuated in both groups in the presence of the metabolic syndrome (MS) demonstrating the presence of endothelial dysfunction. From reference 26, with permission

endothelial progenitor cells which circulate in blood. Recent evidence suggests that there is an inverse cor-

relation between circulating progenitor cells and the risk of cardiovascular events[29]. Importantly many of

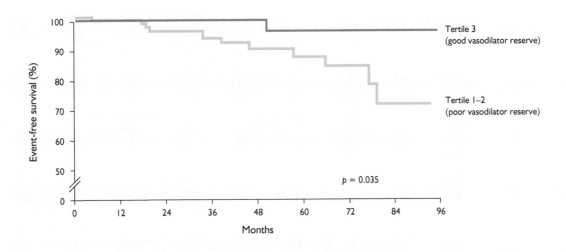

Figure 6.18 Event-free survival for those with the greatest vasodilator reserve (tertile 3) vs. those with the worst vasodilator reserve (tertile 1–2). From reference 27, with permission

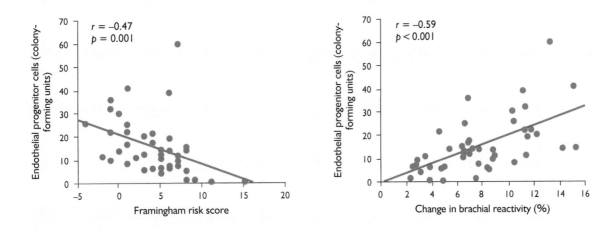

Figure 6.19 Relationship between the reparative capacity (number of endothelial progenitor cells) and the Framingham risk score (a) and flow-mediated dilatation (b). From reference 30, with permission

the factors which contribute to the metabolic syndrome are associated with a reduction in circulating numbers of progenitor cells. Therefore, not only could the metabolic syndrome contribute to endothelial dysfunction but it may also reduce the reparative capacity of the vessel wall.

Hill *et al.* studied the relationship between the reparative capacity (number of endothelial progenitor cells (EPC) colony forming units) and the Framingham risk score and flow-mediated dilatation. They found a significant inverse relationship between EPC and the Framingham risk score and a significant positive relationship between EPC and the flow-mediated dilatation (Figure 6.19). The data strongly support the notion that the presence of reduced numbers of EPC contributes to cardiovascular risk[30].

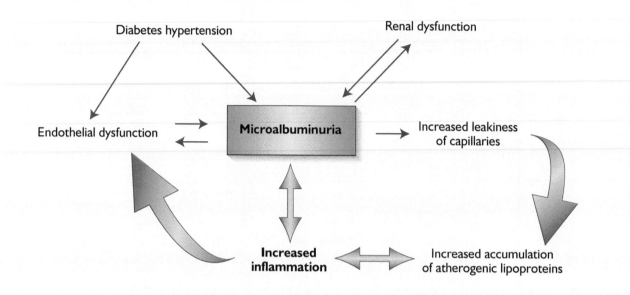

Figure 6.20 Schematic of the postulated multiple mechanisms by which microalbuminuria may be associated with cardiovascular risk

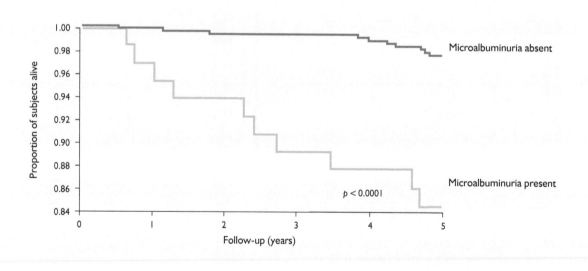

Figure 6.21 Data showing risk of death among subjects with and without microalbuminuria. From reference 32, with permission

MICROALBUMINURIA

Microalbuminuria is defined by the American Diabetes Association as the presence of 30–299 mg of albumin in a 24-hour collection, or an albumin to creatinine ratio of 30–299 µg/mg. The corresponding values for normality or frank macroalbuminuria are < 30 and ≥ 300, respectively. Microalbuminuria is more prevalent among diabetics and in subjects with hypertension; however, some epidemiological data

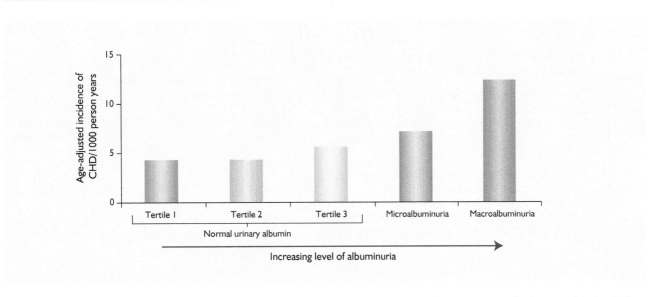

Figure 6.22 Risk of incident CHD in the EPIC-Norfolk Study. These data show the continuum of risk across levels of albumin excretion. Even among 'normoalbuminuric' subjects risk increases across tertiles of albuminuria. It increases further in those with microalbuminuria and is highest among those with macroalbuminuria. The p value for the trend of incidence of CHD events was < 0.0001. From reference 33, with permission

suggest that the prevalence in middle-aged non-diabetics is as high as 10–15%. In a cross-sectional study of approximately 3500 Chinese subjects, the waist-to-hip ratio, systolic and diastolic pressure, serum triglyceride level, fasting plasma glucose, and homeostasis model assessment-insulin resistance (HOMA-IR) were all significantly increased in those subjects with microalbuminuria compared with normal subjects[31]. The prevalence of microalbuminuria was also significantly increased with an incremental rise in the number of components of the metabolic syndrome (p for trend < 0.001). However, the only independent predictors of microalbuminuria were hypertension and hyperglycemia (OR 2.15 and 1.64, respectively).

Mechanisms by which microalbuminuria may be associated with cardiovascular risk are shown in Figure 6.20. Microalbuminuria may be an early renal manifestation of endothelial dysfunction. It may also be a manifestation of increased systemic vascular permeability, which may facilitate an increased flux of atherogenic particles into the arterial wall. These effects may be further accelerated in hypertension or diabetes.

The presence or absence, and the magnitude of albuminuria are powerful predictions of long-term risk (Figures 6.21 and 6.22).

A number of important markers of cardiovascular risk are strongly correlated with microalbuminuria. For example, type 2 diabetic patients with microalbuminuria have more severely impaired coronary endothelium-dependent vasodilatation than those with normoalbuminuria, suggesting a common pathophysiological process for both coronary vasomotor abnormalities and microalbuminuria[34]. In addition, microalbuminuria predicts silent ischemia among diabetics further supporting a pathological role. Furthermore, several cardiovascular risk factors, such as left ventricular mass index and systolic and diastolic dysfunction, are associated with microalbuminuria[35,36].

REFERENCES

1. Ross R. Atherosclerosis – an inflammatory disease [see comments]. N Engl J Med 1999; 340: 115–26

2. Libby P. Current concepts of the pathogenesis of the acute coronary syndromes. Circulation 2001; 104: 365–72

3. Lutgens E, van Suylen RJ, Faber BC, et al. Atherosclerotic plaque rupture: local or systemic process? Arterioscler Thromb Vasc Biol 2003; 23: 2123–30

4. Ridker PM, Rifai N, Stampfer MJ, Hennekens CH. Plasma concentration of interleukin-6 and the risk of future myocardial infarction among apparently healthy men. Circulation 2000; 101: 1767–72

5. Pradhan AD, Manson JE, Rossouw JE, et al. Inflammatory biomarkers, hormone replacement therapy, and incident coronary heart disease: prospective analysis from the Women's Health Initiative observational study. JAMA 2002; 288: 980–7

6. Ray KK, Cannon CP, Cairns R, et al. Relationship between uncontrolled risk factors and C-reactive protein levels in patients receiving standard or intensive statin therapy for acute coronary syndromes in the PROVE IT-TIMI 22 trial. J Am Coll Cardiol 2005; 46: 1417–24

7. Rohde LE, Hennekens CH, Ridker PM. Survey of C-reactive protein and cardiovascular risk factors in apparently healthy men. Am J Cardiol 1999; 84: 1018–22

8. Ridker PM, Buring JE, Cook NR, Rifai N. C-reactive protein, the metabolic syndrome, and risk of incident cardiovascular events: an 8-year follow-up of 14 719 initially healthy American women. Circulation 2003; 107: 391–7

9. Yeh ET. CRP as a mediator of disease. Circulation 2004; 109 (21 Suppl 1): II11–114

10. Ridker PM, Glynn RJ, Hennekens CH. C-reactive protein adds to the predictive value of total and HDL cholesterol in determining risk of first myocardial infarction. Circulation 1998; 97: 2007–11

11. Ridker PM, Hennekens CH, Buring JE, Rifai N. C-reactive protein and other markers of inflammation in the prediction of cardiovascular disease in women. N Engl J Med 2000; 342: 836–43

12. Koenig W, Sund M, Frohlich M, et al. C-reactive protein, a sensitive marker of inflammation, predicts future risk of coronary heart disease in initially healthy middle-aged men: results from the MONICA (Monitoring Trends and Determinants in Cardiovascular Disease) Augsburg Cohort Study, 1984–1992. Circulation 1999; 99: 237–42

13. Folsom AR, Aleksic N, Catellier D, et al. C-reactive protein and incident coronary heart disease in the Atherosclerosis Risk In Communities (ARIC) study. Am Heart J 2002; 144: 233–8

14. Ridker PM, Wilson PW, Grundy SM. Should C-reactive protein be added to metabolic syndrome and to assessment of global cardiovascular risk? Circulation 2004; 109: 2818–25

15. Albert MA, Danielson E, Rifai N, Ridker PM. Effect of statin therapy on C-reacvtive protein levels: the pravastatin inflammation/CRP evaluation (PRINCE): a randomized trail and cohort study. JAMA 2001; 286: 64–70

16. Kohler HP, Grant PJ. Plasminogen-activator inhibitor type 1 and coronary artery disease. N Engl J Med 2000; 342: 1792–801

17. Ridker PM, Rifai N, Rose L, et al. Comparison of C-reactive protein and low-density lipoprotein cholesterol levels in the prediction of first cardiovascular events. N Engl J Med 2002; 347: 1557–65

18. Sattar N, Gaw A, Scherbakova O, et al. Metabolic syndrome with and without C-reactive protein as a predictor of coronary heart disease and diabetes in the West of Scotland Coronary Prevention Study. Circulation 2003; 108: 414–19

19. Os I, Nordby G. Hypertension and the metabolic cardiovascular syndrome: special reference to premenopausal women. J Cardiovasc Pharmacol 1992; 20 (Suppl 8): S15–21

20. Sakkinen PA, Wahl P, Cushman M, et al. Clustering of procoagulation, inflammation, and fibrinolysis variables with metabolic factors in insulin resistance syndrome. Am J Epidemiol 2000; 152: 897–907

21. Svendsen OL, Hassager C, Christiansen C, et al. Plasminogen activator inhibitor-1, tissue-type plasminogen activator, and fibrinogen: effect of dieting with or without exercise in overweight postmenopausal women. Arterioscler Thromb Vasc Biol 1996; 16: 381–5

22. Skurk T, Hauner H. Obesity and impaired fibrinolysis: role of adipose production of plasminogen activator inhibitor-1. Int J Obes Relat Metab Disord 2004; 28: 1357–64

23. Juhan-Vague I, Thompson SG, Jespersen J. Involvement of the hemostatic system in the insulin resistance syndrome. A study of 1500 patients with angina pectoris. The ECAT Angina Pectoris Study Group. Arterioscler Thromb 1993; 13: 1865–73

24. Meade TW, Ruddock V, Stirling Y, et al. Fibrinolytic activity, clotting factors, and long-term incidence of ischaemic heart disease in the Northwick Park Heart Study. Lancet 1993; 342: 1076–9

25. Thogersen AM, Jansson JH, Boman K, et al. High plasminogen activator inhibitor and tissue plasminogen activator levels in plasma precede a first acute myocardial infarction in both men and women: evidence for the fibrinolytic system as an independent primary risk factor. Circulation 1998; 98: 2241–7

26. Lteif AA, Han K, Mather KJ. Obesity, insulin resistance, and the metabolic syndrome: determinants of endothelial dysfunction in whites and blacks. Circulation 2005; 112: 32–8

27. Halcox JP, Schenke WH, Zalos G, et al. Prognostic value of coronary vascular endothelial dysfunction. Circulation 2002; 106: 653–8

28. Suwaidi JA, Hamasaki S, Higano ST, et al. Long-term follow-up of patients with mild coronary artery disease and endothelial dysfunction. Circulation 2000; 101: 948–54

29. Schmidt-Lucke CL, Rossig S, Fichtlscherer M, et al. Reduced number of circulating endothelial progenitor cells predicts future cardiovascular events: proof of concept for the clinical importance of endogenous vascular repair. Circulation 2005; 111: 2981–7

30. Hill JM, Zalos G, Halcox JP, et al. Circulating endothelial progenitor cells, vascular function, and cardiovascular risk. N Engl J Med 2003; 348: 593–600

31. Li Q, Jia WP, Lu JQ, et al. [Relationship between the prevalence of microalbuminuria and components of metabolic syndrome in Shanghai]. Zhonghua Liu Xing Bing Xue Za Zhi 2004; 25: 65–8

32. Jager A, Kostense PJ, Ruhe HG, et al. Microalbuminuria and peripheral arterial disease are independent predictors of cardiovascular and all-cause mortality, especially among hypertensive subjects: five-year follow-up of the Hoorn Study. Arterioscler Thromb Vasc Biol 1999; 19: 617–24

33. Yuyun MF, Khaw KT, Luben R, et al. A prospective study of microalbuminuria and incident coronary heart disease and its prognostic significance in a British population: the EPIC-Norfolk study. Am J Epidemiol 2004; 159: 284–93

34. Cosson E, Pham I, Valensi P, et al. Impaired coronary endothelium-dependent vasodilation is associated with microalbuminuria in patients with type 2 diabetes and angiographically normal coronary arteries. Diabetes Care 2006; 29: 107–12

35. Dell'omo G, Giorgi D, Di Bello V, et al. Blood pressure independent association of microalbuminuria and left ventricular hypertrophy in hypertensive men. J Intern Med 2003; 254: 76–84

36. Liu JE, Robbins DC, Palmieri V, et al. Association of albuminuria with systolic and diastolic left ventricular dysfunction in type 2 diabetes: the Strong Heart Study. J Am Coll Cardiol 2003; 41: 2022–8

7 Clinical outcomes of patients with cardiometabolic risk factors

INTRODUCTION

Despite major advances in prevention and management, cardiovascular disease continues to be the leading cause of death in the United States. Although significant efforts have been made to reduce the burden of cardiovascular risk, the prevalence of risk factors continues to be high within the US population. As our understanding of the pathophysiology of cardiovascular disease grows, new risk factors such as the metabolic syndrome and markers of inflammation including C-reactive protein (CRP) are being recognized. These newly defined risk factors identify additional patients at increased risk of cardiovascular events that may not have been previously recognized. Furthermore, the majority of patients now present with multiple risk factors that may have a synergistic effect on overall cardiovascular risk. The term 'metabolic syndrome' has been used to describe the combination of modifiable risk factors that identifies patients at an elevated risk for future cardiovascular events. Several risk factors in the metabolic syndrome also identify patients at risk for developing type 2 diabetes mellitus.

Table 7.1 lists the numerous cardiometabolic risk factors. This chapter will review the risk of cardiovascular complications and outcomes associated with each of these cardiometabolic risk factors.

HYPERTENSION

Hypertension continues to be one of the most prevalent and treatable components of the cardiometabolic syndrome. A recent review of the National Health and Nutrition Examination Survey (NHANES) suggests that an estimated 58.4 million Americans have high blood pressure requiring therapy[1]. Worldwide, the prevalence of hypertension has been estimated to be as high as 1 billion people with 7.1 million deaths per year related to its complications[2]. In the US, hypertension continues to be underdiagnosed and undertreated with approximately 30% of patients remaining unaware of their hypertension, 40% of patients not receiving any treatment, and another two-thirds with blood pressure above 140/90[3]. The prevalence of hypertension increases with age with approximately 75% of patients aged 70 or older demonstrating high blood pressure[4]. The recent Seventh Report of the Joint National Committee on Prevention, Detection, Evaluation, and Treatment of High Blood Pressure

Table 7.1 Cardiometabolic risk factors

Hypertension

Abdominal adiposity

Low HDL cholesterol

High LDL cholesterol

Hypertriglyceridemia

Impaired glucose tolerance, impaired fasting glucose, insulin resistance, and diabetes

Metabolic syndrome

Smoking

Inflammatory markers including C-reactive protein

Table 7.2 Classification of blood pressure in adults. From reference 3, with permission

BP classification	SBP (mmHg)	DBP (mmHg)
Normal	< 120	and < 80
Prehypertension	120–139	or 80–89
Stage 1 hypertension	140–159	or 90–99
Stage 2 hypertension	≥ 160	or ≥ 100

BP, blood pressure; SBP, systolic blood pressure; DBP, diastolic blood pressure

Table 7.3 Cardiovascular complications of hypertension

Coronary artery disease
Left ventricular systolic dysfunction leading to congestive heart failure
Left ventricular diastolic dysfunction leading to congestive heart failure
Left ventricular hypertrophy
Atrial fibrillation
Cerebrovascular disease
Peripheral arterial disease

(JNC VII) proposed new definitions for hypertension and prehypertension (Table 7.2)[3].

Because of its increasing prevalence and wide-reaching effects on morbidity and mortality, hypertension continues to be a crucial target in cardiovascular risk reduction. Many consider hypertension to be the dominant risk factor for premature onset cardiovascular disease because it is more common than smoking, dyslipidemia, and diabetes[5]. The cardiovascular complications of hypertension include coronary artery disease, left ventricular systolic and diastolic dysfunction leading to congestive heart failure, left ventricular hypertrophy, atrial fibrillation, cerebrovascular disease, and peripheral arterial disease (Table 7.3). The World Health Organization has suggested that poorly controlled blood pressure may be responsible for up to 62% of cerebrovascular disease and 49% of coronary artery disease[3]. The Framingham Heart Study has demonstrated that the first manifestations of the cardiovascular complications of hypertension tend to be coronary artery disease in men and stroke in women[6]. The risk of cardiovascular events has been shown to increase according to the degree of hypertension, and this relationship appears to strengthen with advancing age[7]. A recent study revealed that both increasing severity of systolic and diastolic hypertension correlated with risk of all-cause and cardiovascular mortality regardless of patient age, although a J-shaped curve was suggested for diastolic blood pressure at advanced ages (Figure 7.1)[8]. Data from observational studies have demonstrated a linear relationship between risk of death from both ischemic heart disease and stroke and increasing levels of systolic and diastolic blood pressure in all age groups ranging from 40 to 89 years old (Figures 7.2 and 7.3)[9]. Before JNC VII, patients with 'prehypertension' or blood pressures ranging from 120 to 139 mmHg systolic and/or 80 to 89 mmHg diastolic were not widely recognized as a population at increased risk for cardiovascular events. However, long-term follow-up data from the Framingham Heart Study have demonstrated a two-fold increase in the relative risk of cardiovascular events among patients with blood pressures of 130–139/85–89 mmHg (Figure 7.4)[10].

In addition to these cardiovascular complications, hypertension is also an important cause of chronic kidney disease (Figures 7.5 and 7.6) and may be a predisposing factor in the development of type 2 diabetes mellitus. One study demonstrated that patients with hypertension were nearly 2.5 times more likely to develop type 2 diabetes than those without hypertension[12]. In the Heart Outcomes Prevention Evaluation (HOPE) study, patients at high risk for cardiovascular events receiving the antihypertensive ramipril (an angiotensin-converting enzyme inhibitor) had a significant reduction in the relative risk of developing diabetes compared with those receiving placebo[13]. It remains unclear whether hypertension itself is a risk factor for the development of diabetes or if it is associated with other factors such as obesity that may contribute to insulin resistance and diabetes. Furthermore, the reduction in the diagnosis of new diabetes among patients receiving ramipril in the HOPE study may be related to intrinsic properties of the medication itself rather than its blood pressure-lowering effects, as other antihypertensives have not been shown to reduce the incidence of diabetes. Frequently coexistent, hypertension and diabetes in combination have a particularly potent effect on the risk of cardiovascular disease. In the Systolic Hypertension in the Elderly Program (SHEP)

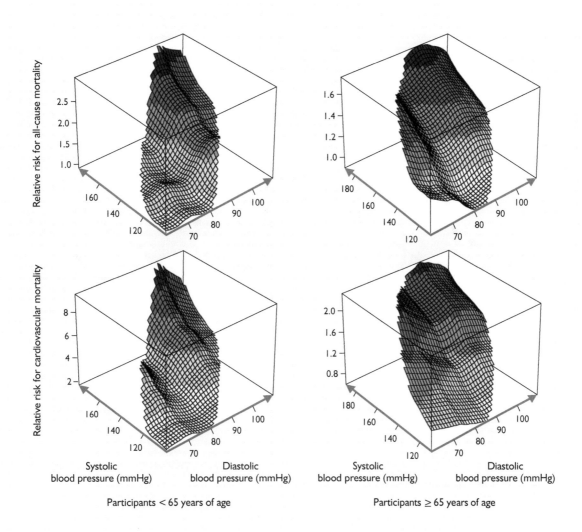

Figure 7.1 Risk surfaces for all-cause and cardiovascular mortality as a function of systolic and diastolic blood pressure by age groups of <65 or ≥65 years old. The surfaces demonstrate the relative risk for all-cause and cardiovascular mortality for combinations of systolic and diastolic blood pressure. From reference 8, with permission

study, hypertensive patients with diabetes receiving blood pressure-lowering therapy with low-dose diuretics demonstrated twice the absolute risk reduction in cardiovascular events compared with hypertensive patients without diabetes[14]. In the Systolic Hypertension in Europe (Syst Eur) Trial, the same degree of blood pressure-lowering was associated with a 76% risk reduction in cardiovascular mortality among diabetic patients receiving antihypertensive therapy compared with a 13% reduction among non-diabetic patients[15]. These studies suggest that patients with diabetes and hypertension are at a significantly

increased risk of cardiovascular events compared with non-diabetics with hypertension and that aggressive antihypertensive therapy should be pursued in these high-risk patients. Even prehypertensive patients with diabetes demonstrate a significantly higher risk of cardiovascular events compared with non-diabetic prehypertensive patients[16].

A growing body of evidence has established hypertension as one of the most important modifiable risk factors for cardiovascular disease and an integral component of the cardiometabolic syndrome. Hypertension significantly augments the risk of cardiovascular

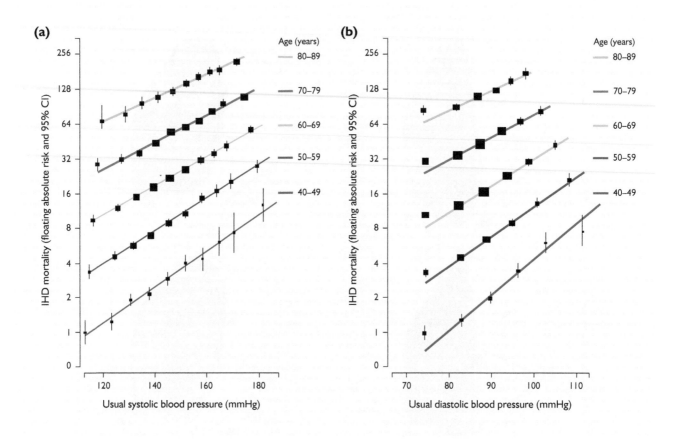

Figure 7.2 Ischemic heart disease mortality rate in each decade of age versus usual systolic (a) and diastolic (b) blood pressure at the start of that decade. From reference 9, with permission

events when combined with other cardiometabolic risk factors such as diabetes.

OBESITY AND ABDOMINAL ADIPOSITY

The problem of obesity has reached epidemic proportions in the majority of developed nations worldwide. The World Health Organization (WHO) has reported that over 1 billion adults worldwide meet the definition for overweight (body mass index (BMI) of greater than 25 kg/m^2) and at least 300 million adults meet criteria for clinical obesity (BMI of greater than 30 kg/m^2)[17]. Obesity is associated with a myriad of medical conditions including coronary artery disease, peripheral arterial disease, cerebrovascular disease, congestive heart failure, the metabolic syndrome, hypertension, insulin resistance, type 2 diabetes mellitus,

dyslipidemia, obstructive sleep apnea, liver disease, and degenerative joint disease. A subset of obese patients demonstrate abdominal obesity or adiposity which is defined by increasing waist circumference, sagittal abdominal diameter, and waist-to-hip ratio. Waist circumference and sagittal abdominal diameter have been shown to correlate best with intra-abdominal adiposity which is a risk factor for cardiovascular disease as well as for dyslipidemia and diabetes[18]. The definition for abdominal adiposity varies between different ethnic populations as well as within the current literature. A recent study revealed that 36.9% of men and 55.1% of women in the US met the definition of abdominal adiposity based on high-risk waist circumference (waist circumference of greater than 102 cm in men and greater than 88 cm in women)[19].

Overall obesity has been identified as a major risk factor for cardiovascular events and mortality. A

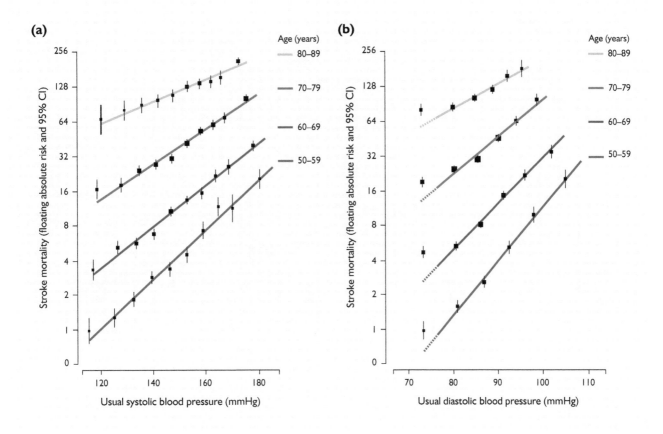

Figure 7.3 Stroke mortality rate in each decade of age versus usual systolic (a) and diastolic (b) blood pressure at the start of that decade. From reference 9, with permission

prospective study of over 1 million adults in the US evaluated the relationship between BMI and cardiovascular mortality as well as all-cause mortality[20]. The risk of death from cardiovascular disease as well as all causes was noted to increase progressively over the range of overweight to clinically obese patients regardless of age or sex (Figure 7.7)[20]. One study demonstrated that risk factors for coronary artery disease such as low HDL cholesterol levels, systolic blood pressure, triglycerides, glucose, and serum total cholesterol often cluster with obesity[21]. The study also demonstrated that a 2.25 kg weight reduction was associated with a 48% reduction in the sum of risk factors for coronary artery disease in man and a similar 40% reduction in women[21]. A recent study investigated the relationship between being overweight or obese at 40 years of age and life expectancy[22]. Overweight and obesity were both strongly associated with

large decreases in life expectancy, even among patients who were non-smokers (Figure 7.8)[22]. Another recent study investigated the impact of BMI and measures of abdominal adiposity including waist circumference and waist-to-hip ratio on the prognosis of patients with stable cardiovascular disease who had been enrolled in the Heart Outcomes Prevention Evaluation (HOPE) study[23]. When compared with the first tertile, the third tertile of BMI was associated with a 20% increase in the relative risk of myocardial infarction[23]. The third tertile of waist circumference was associated with a 23% increase in the relative risk of myocardial infarction, a 38% increase in the relative risk of heart failure, and a 17% relative increase in total mortality when compared with the first tertile[23]. Patients within the third tertile of waist-to-hip ratio demonstrated a 24% increased relative risk of cardiovascular death, a 20% increased relative risk of

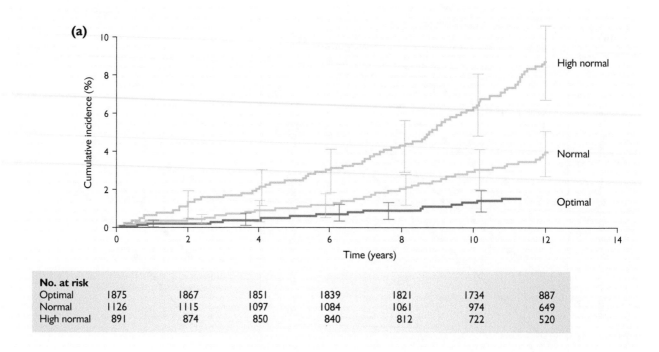

No. at risk

Optimal	1875	1867	1851	1839	1821	1734	887
Normal	1126	1115	1097	1084	1061	974	649
High normal	891	874	850	840	812	722	520

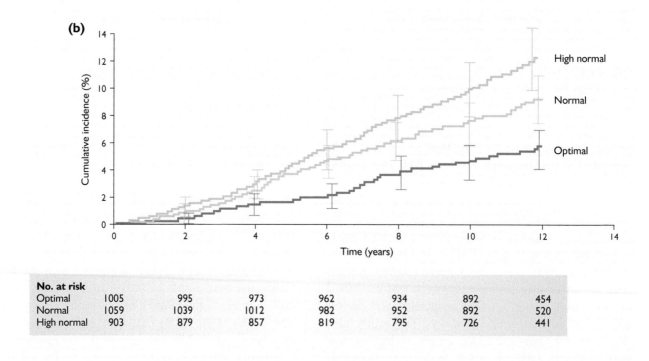

No. at risk

Optimal	1005	995	973	962	934	892	454
Normal	1059	1039	1012	982	952	892	520
High normal	903	879	857	819	795	726	441

Figure 7.4 Impact of high-normal blood pressure on the cumulative incidence of cardiovascular disease among women (a) and men (b). Optimal blood pressure is defined as a systolic blood pressure of < 120 mmHg and diastolic blood pressure of < 80 mmHg. Normal blood pressure is defined as a systolic blood pressure of 120–129 mmHg or a diastolic blood pressure of 80–84 mmHg. High-normal blood pressure is defined as a systolic blood pressure of 130–139 mmHg and a diastolic blood pressure of 85–89 mmHg. From reference 10, with permission

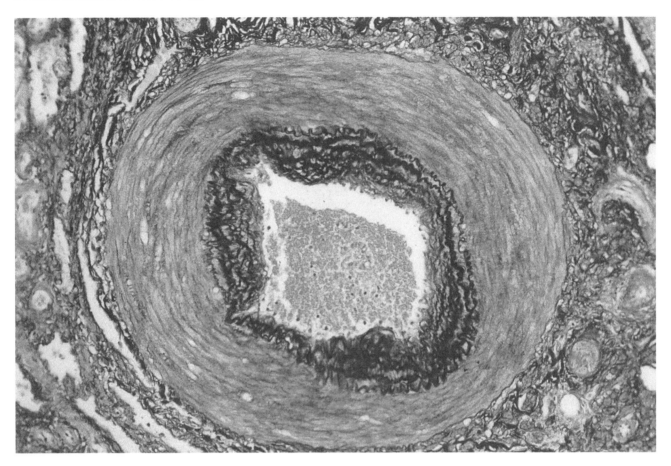

Figure 7.5 Histology showing a renal artery in the early stages of established hypertension showing medial hypertrophy and intimal thickening causing an increase in wall: lumen ratio. Intimal thickening is a result of an increase in collagen and elastic (black-staining) matrix proteins (elastica van Gieson). From reference 11, with permission

myocardial infarction, and a 32% relative increase in total mortality[23]. Based on this study, obesity and, more importantly, abdominal adiposity appear to correlate with a worse prognosis among patients with stable cardiovascular disease.

Like obesity, abdominal adiposity is associated with other major cardiovascular risk factors including low high-density lipoprotein (HDL) cholesterol levels, high low-density lipoprotein (LDL) cholesterol, high triglyceride levels, diabetes, and hypertension. While abdominal adiposity is an important independent risk factor for cardiovascular disease, it is also a component of the diagnostic criteria for the metabolic syndrome. An improved understanding of adipocyte pathophysiology has given rise to the concept of adipose tissue as an endocrine organ with widespread effects on lipid metabolism, glucose control, vascular function, and atherosclerosis[24]. In the INTERHEART study which

comprised 52 countries on every inhabited continent, the relationship between multiple cardiovascular risk factors and the incidence of myocardial infarction was evaluated[25]. Abdominal adiposity and other major risk factors including dyslipidemia, smoking, hypertension, diabetes, and psychosocial factors were all significantly associated with an increased incidence of myocardial infarction[25]. In a prospective study of women participating in the Nurses' Health Study, the relationship of waist circumference and waist-to-hip ratio to the incidence of coronary artery disease was evaluated[26]. Greater waist circumference and increased waist-to-hip ratio were found to be independently associated with a significant age-adjusted increase in coronary artery disease[26]. A recent study, utilizing the data from the Paris Prospective Study I, investigated the relationship between overall obesity and abdominal obesity on the risk of sudden cardiac death among men

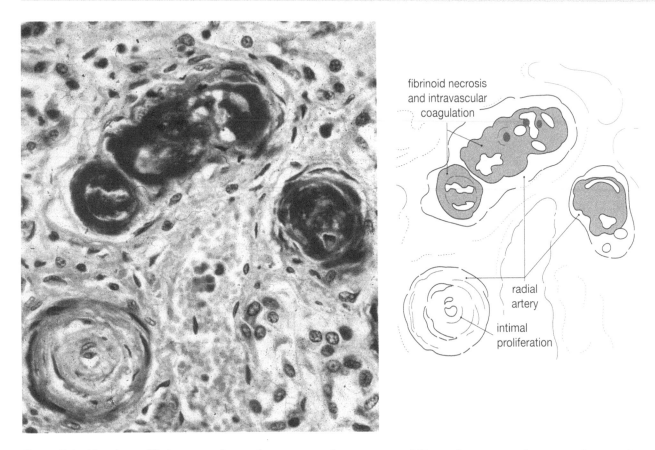

Figure 7.6 Histology of kidney in malignant hypertension showing areas of fibrinoid necrosis and intravascular coagulation. The remaining terminal interlobular artery shows 'onion-skin' proliferative enarteritis probably as a healing response to acute injury (Masson trichrome). From reference 11, with permission

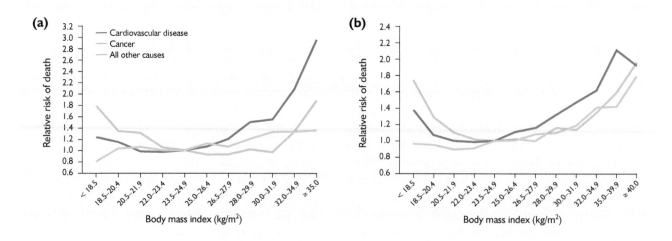

Figure 7.7 Multivariate relative risk of death from cardiovascular disease, cancer, and all other causes among men (a) and women (b) who were never smokers and had no history of disease at the start of the study according to body mass index. From reference 20, with permission

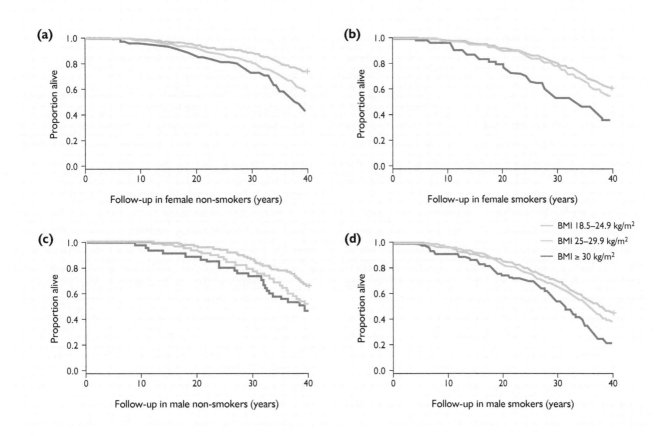

Figure 7.8 Kaplan–Meier survival estimates for body mass index groups for female non-smokers (a), female smokers (b), male non-smokers (c), and male smokers (d). BMI, body mass index. From reference 22, with permission

without history of ischemic heart disease[27]. Increasing sagittal abdominal diameter was shown to correlate with proportional increases in the risk of sudden cardiac death independent of BMI (Figure 7.9)[27]. In addition, patients in the fifth quintile of sagittal abdominal diameter were 2.6 times more likely to develop a fatal myocardial infarction compared with those in the first quintile[27]. Based on these data, abdominal adiposity has emerged as an independent and important cardiovascular risk factor.

Overall obesity and abdominal adiposity are also associated with an increased risk of hyperglycemia, insulin resistance, and overt diabetes. Intra-abdominal adiposity has been shown to lead to impaired pancreatic beta cell function[28]. Furthermore, the extent of intra-abdominal adiposity has been shown to correlate strongly with increasing degrees of insulin resistance[29]. A recent study compared BMI as a measure of overall obesity with waist circumference and waist-to-hip

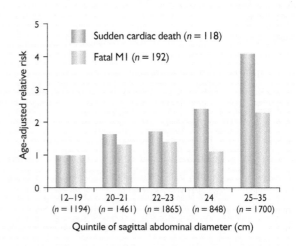

Figure 7.9 Age-adjusted relative risk of sudden cardiac death and fatal myocardial infarction by quintile of sagittal abdominal diameter. From reference 27, with permission

ratio as measures of abdominal adiposity as risk factors for the development of type 2 diabetes[30]. While both overall obesity and abdominal adiposity were strong independent risk factors for the development of type 2 diabetes, BMI and waist circumference were better predictors than waist-to-hip ratio[30]. Another study compared the effect of lifestyle modifications including at least a 7% weight reduction and 150 minutes per week of physical activity with that of metformin in patients at an elevated risk for developing type 2 diabetes[31]. The lifestyle intervention group demonstrated a 58% reduction in the incidence of type 2 diabetes compared with placebo, while metformin was associated with a 31% reduction[31]. While this study suggested that lifestyle modifications lead to a greater reduction in the incidence of type 2 diabetes than metformin, it also demonstrated the important role that obesity plays in the pathogenesis of diabetes.

Although overall obesity has been a well-established risk factor for cardiovascular disease and diabetes, abdominal adiposity has recently emerged as an important and independent risk factor. An assessment for abdominal adiposity, such as determination of the waist circumference, in addition to estimation of the BMI as a measure of overall obesity should be performed in the evaluation of each patient's overall cardiometabolic risk.

LOW HIGH-DENSITY LIPOPROTEIN LEVELS

While much of the current focus of therapy for dyslipidemia centers on management of high LDL cholesterol, low HDL cholesterol levels have also been established as a major cardiovascular risk factor. In fact, the pattern of low HDL cholesterol levels with normal LDL cholesterol levels appears to represent a significant percentage of patients with coronary artery disease when compared with isolated high LDL cholesterol[32]. Low HDL cholesterol levels are also an important part of the criteria for the metabolic syndrome, which includes a constellation of other risk factors that place patients at a markedly increased risk for cardiovascular events. Low HDL cholesterol is defined by the Third Report of the National Cholesterol Education Program (NCEP) Expert Panel on Detection, Evaluation, and Treatment of High Blood Cholesterol

in Adults (Adult Treatment Panel III (ATP III)) as a serum level of less than 40 mg/dL[33].

As an independent risk factor, low HDL cholesterol levels have consistently been associated with an increased risk of cardiovascular disease. In the Framingham Heart Study, patients with the highest levels of HDL cholesterol demonstrated the lowest incidence of coronary artery disease in long-term follow-up[34]. In another study from the Framingham Heart Study, patients with HDL cholesterol levels within the 80th percentile demonstrated half of the risk of developing coronary artery disease compared with those in the 20th percentile[35]. An analysis of men enrolled in the Physicians' Health Study evaluated the contribution of low HDL cholesterol levels to the risk of myocardial infarction[36]. Low HDL cholesterol levels correlated with a significantly increased risk for myocardial infarction and this relationship was even more pronounced in patients with lower total cholesterol levels[36]. A recent study compared the effects of LDL cholesterol and HDL cholesterol on overall mortality with the risk of cardiovascular disease among a group of advanced elderly patients[37]. Cardiovascular disease was the leading cause of death among the study patients and this risk mortality was similar across all tertiles of LDL cholesterol[37]. However, a low HDL cholesterol level correlated with a significantly increased risk of mortality from both myocardial infarction and stroke[37] (Figure 7.10). Low HDL cholesterol levels have also been associated with a significantly increased risk of restenosis after percutaneous transluminal coronary angioplasty (PTCA)[38]. Another study demonstrated that decreasing levels of HDL cholesterol correlated with a significant increase in the number of vessels affected with coronary artery disease as well as with the incidence of left main coronary artery disease regardless of patient age or gender[39]. Among patients with known coronary artery disease, low levels of HDL cholesterol have also been shown to be independently associated with a significantly increased relative risk of recurrent cardiovascular events when compared with patients with desirable levels[40].

Based on these data, patients should be assessed for low HDL cholesterol as both an independent risk factor for cardiovascular disease and an important component of the metabolic syndrome. Although high LDL cholesterol levels continue to be an important modifiable risk factor, multiple studies suggest that

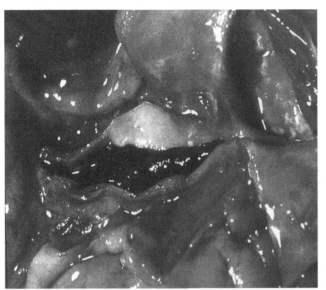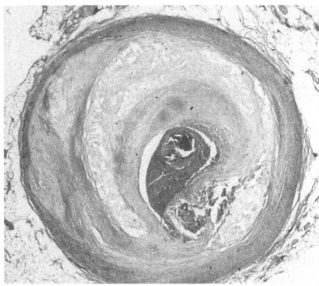

Figure 7.10 Recent thombus can be seen at the origin of the right coronary artery close to aorta (left). Histology showing a severely atheromatous coronary artery (right) shows residual media (deep pink-staining). The artery is narrowed by atheromatous plaque comprising a mixture of pale fibrous tissue and clear lipid material. The plaque cap has ruptured, causing hemorrhage into the plaque and thrombosis of the lumen (H & E). From reference 11, with permission

Table 7.4 NCEP ATP III classification of LDL cholesterol in 2002. From reference 33, with permission

Classification	LDL cholesterol (mg/dL)
Optimal	< 100
Near or above optimal	100–129
Borderline high	130–159
High	160–189
Very high	≥ 190

New studies since 2002 may lead to further refinement in classification of LDL levels

HDL cholesterol should be an important target in the reduction of cardiometabolic risk.

HIGH LOW-DENSITY LIPOPROTEIN LEVELS

High LDL cholesterol levels have gained increasing importance over the past several years not only as a major cardiovascular risk factor, but also as a crucial target in primary and secondary prevention. The NCEP ATP III classifies LDL cholesterol levels of less than 100 mg/dL as optimal, 100–129 mg/dL as near or above optimal, 130–159 mg/dL as borderline high, 160–189 mg/dL as high, and greater than or equal to 190 mg/dL as very high (Table 7.4)[33]. These classifications reflect the observation that patients with LDL cholesterol levels that were previously thought to be 'normal' or 'average' still demonstrate an increased risk for cardiovascular events when compared with patients with lower levels (Figure 7.11).

Elevated levels of LDL cholesterol have been demonstrated in numerous studies to be associated with a significantly increased risk of cardiovascular events including coronary artery disease. In a study of 2541 white men with and without coronary artery disease, the relationships between levels of total, HDL, and LDL cholesterol and risk of death from cardiovascular and coronary artery disease were evaluated[42]. Among patients with evidence of cardiovascular disease at baseline, a higher level of LDL cholesterol correlated with an increased risk of death from coronary artery disease[42]. LDL cholesterol levels were also shown to be significant predictors of death from cardiovascular and coronary artery disease among patients without a history of cardiovascular disease[42]. Data from the Framingham Heart Study have also demonstrated that LDL cholesterol is an effective predictor of coronary artery disease risk in both men and women[43]. The Lipid Research Clinics Coronary

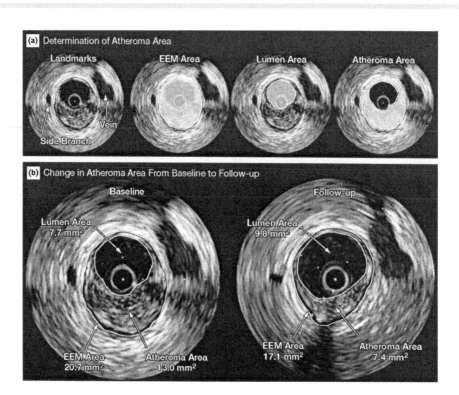

Figure 7.11   (a) Atheroma area is calculated by subtracting the lumen area from the area of the external elastic membrane (EEM). (b) Patient randomized to 80 mg of atorvastatin. There is substantial reduction in atheroma area (from 13.0 to 7.4 mm^2). A lesser increase in lumen area is noted (from 7.7 to 9.8 mm^2). See video at http://jama.com/cgi/content/full/291/9/1071/DC1. From reference 41, with permission

Primary Prevention Trial evaluated the efficacy of lowering total and LDL cholesterol with cholestyramine in the reduction of coronary artery disease risk among asymptomatic men[44]. The cholesterol-lowering group demonstrated an average reduction in LDL cholesterol of 20.3% which was associated with a 19% reduction in the primary end point of risk of death from coronary artery disease and risk of non-fatal myocardial infarction[44]. In addition, the cholesterol-lowering group experienced reductions in the incidence of positive exercise stress tests, anginal episodes, and coronary artery bypass surgery[44]. The study also demonstrated a 19% relative risk reduction in coronary artery disease with each 11% reduction in LDL cholesterol level[45]. The West of Scotland Coronary Prevention Study (WOSCOPS) evaluated the effect of lipid-lowering with pravastatin among patients with hyperlipidemia and no history of coronary artery disease[46]. The pravastatin treatment group experienced a 26% reduction in LDL cholesterol compared with no change in the placebo group[46]. Treatment with pravastatin was associated with a 31% relative risk reduction

in coronary events including non-fatal myocardial infarction or death from coronary artery disease[46]. Significant risk reductions in non-fatal myocardial infarction, death from coronary heart disease, and death from all cardiovascular causes were also observed[46]. In the Air Force/Texas Coronary Atherosclerosis Prevention Study (AFCAPS/TexCAPS), lovastatin was compared with placebo in the prevention of first acute major coronary events defined as fatal and non-fatal myocardial infarction, unstable angina, or sudden cardiac death among patients without known cardiovascular disease and 'average' cholesterol levels (mean LDL cholesterol level was 150 mg/dL)[47]. After average follow-up of more than 5 years, lovastatin decreased LDL cholesterol levels by 25% and led to significant reductions in the incidence of first acute major coronary events, myocardial infarction, unstable angina, coronary revascularization procedures, coronary events, and cardiovascular events[47].

Several large randomized controlled trials have evaluated the effect of LDL cholesterol lowering with 3-hydroxy-3-methyl-glutaryl-coenzyme A reductase

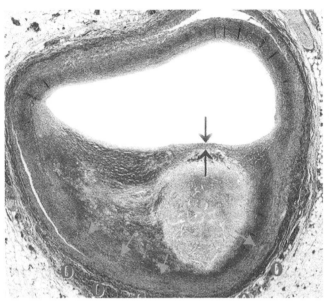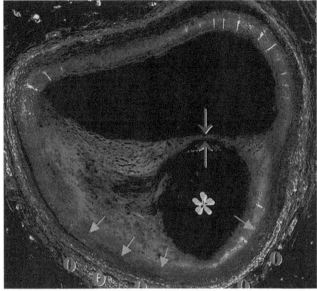

Figure 7.12   Molecular and structural targets for imaging. Cross-section of a coronary artery containing plaque assumed to be rupture-prone. Potential targets for imaging are highlighted. They comprise: the large lipid-rich necrotic core (orange asterisk), thin fibrous cap (blue arrows), expansive remodeling (green arrow), and vasa vasorum and neovascularization (red open circles). From reference 48, with permission

inhibitors (statins) in patients with known cardiovascular disease and 'average' serum levels on the risk of cardiovascular events, showing a benefit in preventing plaque rupture (Figures 7.12 and 7.13).

In the Cholesterol and Recurrent Events (CARE) Trial, 4159 patients with myocardial infarction and a mean LDL cholesterol level of 139 mg/dL were randomized to LDL lowering with pravastatin or placebo[50]. The pravastatin therapy group demonstrated a 32% reduction in LDL cholesterol level which was associated with a 24% relative risk reduction in fatal coronary events or non-fatal myocardial infarction[50]. Significant reductions in the need for coronary artery bypass surgery, coronary angioplasty, and stroke were also noted in the treatment group[50]. Of note, the risk reduction in coronary events was greatest in the patients with the highest pretreatment LDL cholesterol levels[50]. The Heart Protection Study evaluated the effects of simvastatin on mortality as well as fatal and non-fatal vascular events among patients with known cardiovascular disease or diabetes[51]. A significant decrease in mortality largely attributable to an 18% reduction in coronary death rate was noted in the simvastatin treatment group[51]. The study also demonstrated significant reductions in non-fatal myocardial

infarction and coronary death, non-fatal or fatal stroke, and coronary or non-coronary revascularization[51]. Importantly, these reductions in cardiovascular events were observed even in patients with LDL cholesterol levels below 116 mg/dL and even below 100 mg/dL suggesting that LDL levels considered to be 'average' were still associated with significant cardiovascular risk and that statins may have intrinsic cardioprotective effects in addition to their lipid-lowering effects[51]. In the Pravastatin or Atorvastatin Evaluation and Infection Therapy – Thrombolysis in Myocardial Infarction 22 (PROVE IT-TIMI 22) study, 4162 patients who were hospitalized for acute coronary syndromes (ACS) were randomized to standard therapy with 40 mg of pravastatin daily or intensive LDL-lowering therapy with 80 mg of atorvastatin[52]. The median LDL cholesterol level achieved with standard therapy was 95 mg/dL compared with 62 mg/dL in the intensive LDL-lowering therapy group[52]. A significant 16% relative risk reduction in the primary composite end point of death from any cause, myocardial infarction, documented unstable angina requiring hospitalization, revascularization, and stroke was observed in the intensive LDL-lowering group compared with standard therapy (Figure 7.14)[52]. The A to Z investigators

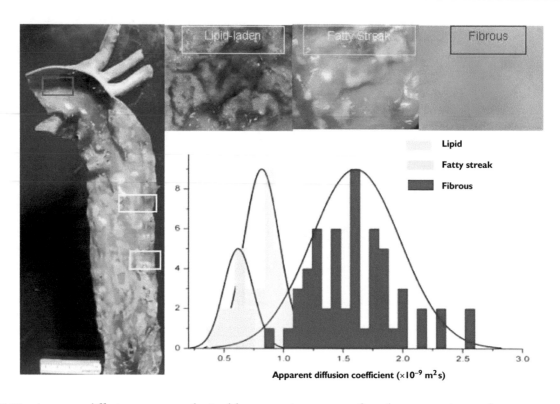

Figure 7.13 Apparent diffusion constants obtained by magnetic resonance from human aortic samples containing normal fibrous tissue, fatty streaks, and complex lipid-laden lesions are seen in photomicrographs. The apparent diffusion constant shows clear difference between the fibrous and lipid-rich tissue, with overlap noted between lipid-rich and fatty streak tissue (studies performed in collaboration with Dr Renu Virmani). From reference 49, with permission

compared an early intensive LDL-lowering regimen of simvastatin 40 mg daily for 1 month followed by 80 mg daily thereafter with a delayed conservative strategy with placebo for 4 months followed by simvastatin 20 mg daily thereafter among patients with ACS[53]. Although no significant difference in the primary composite end point of cardiovascular death, non-fatal myocardial infarction, readmission for ACS, and stroke was noted between the two groups during the first 4 months, a 25% reduction in the risk of the primary end point was observed after the first 4 months through follow-up in the early intensive therapy group[53]. In the randomized controlled Treating to New Targets (TNT) study, the effect of aggressive LDL-lowering with atorvastatin 80 mg daily on cardiovascular events was compared with low-intensity therapy with atorvastatin 10 mg daily among patients with stable coronary artery disease[54]. The mean LDL cholesterol level achieved in the atorvastatin 80 mg group was 77 mg/dL compared with 101 mg/dL in the atorvastatin 10 mg group[54]. A 22% relative risk

reduction in the primary end point of first major cardiovascular event as well as significant reductions in major coronary events, non-fatal myocardial infarction or death from coronary artery disease, and fatal or non-fatal stroke were demonstrated in the atorvastatin 80 mg group (Figure 7.15)[54]. Of note, the atorvastatin 80 mg group experienced a greater incidence of elevated aminotransferase levels than the 10 mg group[54]. Figure 7.16 summarizes the relationship between LDL cholesterol levels and the rate of cardiovascular events among the major secondary prevention trials utilizing statins[54]. The recent Incremental Decrease in End Points Through Aggressive Lipid Lowering (IDEAL) study compared intensive LDL-lowering with atorvastatin 80 mg daily with standard therapy with simvastatin 20 mg daily in the prevention of cardiovascular events among patients with a history of myocardial infarction[55]. During the treatment period, mean LDL cholesterol levels were 81 mg/dL among patients receiving atorvastatin 80 mg daily and 104 mg/dL among patients receiving simvastatin

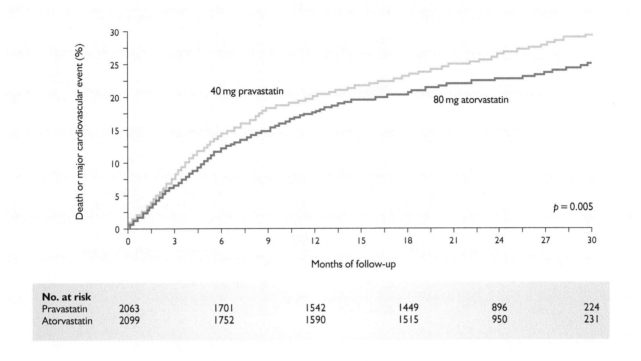

Figure 7.14 Kaplan–Meier estimates comparing the incidence of the primary composite end point of death from any cause or a major cardiovascular event including myocardial infarction, documented unstable angina requiring hospitalization, revascularization, and stroke among the intensive lipid-lowering group (atorvastatin 80 mg daily) and the standard therapy group (pravastatin 40 mg daily) in the PROVE IT-TIMI 22 trial. From reference 52, with permission

20–40 mg daily[55]. Significant reductions in non-fatal acute myocardial infarction, major cardiovascular events including stroke, any coronary event including hospitalization for unstable angina as well as coronary revascularization procedures, and any cardiovascular disease including peripheral arterial disease and non-fatal congestive heart failure were demonstrated in the atorvastatin 80 mg group[55].

The large body of literature supporting the use of LDL-lowering therapy such as statins for the primary and secondary prevention of cardiovascular disease highlights the importance of LDL cholesterol as a significant cardiometabolic risk factor. Risk assessment should include determination of a patient's lipid profile including the LDL cholesterol as well as interpretation of the levels in the context of the patient's other risk factors and the LDL goals suggested by the recent literature and the ATP III.

HYPERTRIGLYCERIDEMIA

Hypertriglyceridemia shares similarities with low HDL cholesterol levels in that it is both an important independent risk factor for cardiovascular disease and part of the criteria for the metabolic syndrome. Hypertriglyceridemia is generally diagnosed when triglyceride levels are elevated above 150 mg/dL[33]. In a meta-analysis of several large prospective trials, the effect of hypertriglyceridemia on the incidence of cardiovascular disease was investigated[56]. Hypertriglyceridemia was associated with nearly a 30% increase in the relative risk of cardiovascular disease among men and a 75% increase among women[56]. Although the relative risk increases attenuated after adjustment for HDL cholesterol levels and other risk factors, a statistically significant increase in risk persisted for both men and women suggesting that hypertriglyceridemia was an independent risk

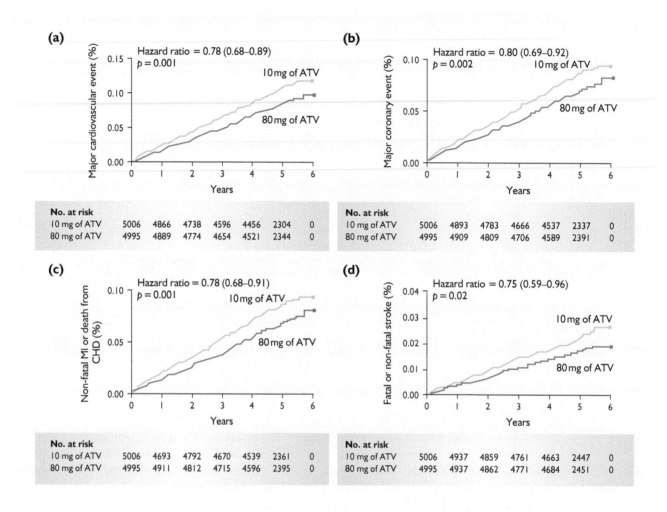

Figure 7.15 Cumulative incidence of a first major cardiovascular event (a), first major coronary event (b), non-fatal myocardial infarction or death from coronary heart disease (c), and fatal or non-fatal stroke (d) in the Treating to New Targets trial. ATV, atorvastatin. From reference 54, with permission

predictor for cardiovascular disease[56]. The Prospective Cardiovascular Munster (PROCAM) Study demonstrated a significant and independent relationship between elevated serum triglyceride levels and major coronary events[57]. A recent study also confirmed that elevated levels of triglycerides were associated with an increased risk of coronary artery disease independent of other lipid abnormalities such as elevated total cholesterol and low HDL cholesterol[58]. These studies suggest that hypertriglyceridemia is an important component of the cardiometabolic syndrome and that triglyceride levels should be determined as part of the cardiovascular risk factor assessment offered to patients.

IMPAIRED GLUCOSE TOLERANCE, IMPAIRED FASTING GLUCOSE, INSULIN RESISTANCE, AND DIABETES

Impaired glucose tolerance, impaired fasting glucose, insulin resistance, and diabetes mellitus represent a spectrum of disorders that is associated with an elevated risk of cardiovascular complications. Impaired glucose tolerance, impaired fasting glucose, and insulin resistance are also risk factors for the development of overt diabetes. Importantly, the NCEP ATP III considers diabetes to be a coronary heart disease risk equivalent, conferring the same risk for coronary events as would be observed in a patient with known coronary

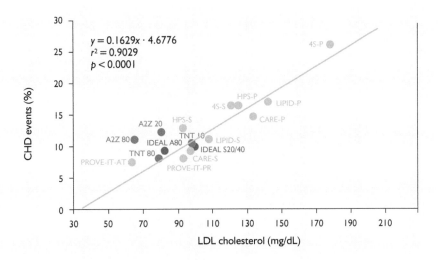

$$y = 0.1629x \cdot 4.6776$$
$$r^2 = 0.9029$$
$$p < 0.0001$$

Figure 7.16 The relationship between cardiovascular event rates and LDL cholesterol levels during statin therapy in major secondary prevention trials. HPS, Health Protection Study; CARE, Cholesterol And Recurrent Events; LIPID, Long-term Intervention with Pravastatin in Ischemic Disease; 4S, Scandinavian Simvastatin Survival Study; TNT, Treating to New Targets. Adapted and updated from reference 54, with permission

artery disease[33]. While diabetes has been a well-established cardiovascular risk factor, impaired glucose tolerance, impaired fasting glucose, and insulin resistance are emerging risk factors that are also associated with the metabolic syndrome as well as the development of overt diabetes. In general, impaired glucose tolerance is determined with an oral glucose tolerance test, impaired fasting glucose is detected by serum glucose after a fast, and insulin resistance is suggested by an elevated fasting serum insulin level.

A study of three European cohorts from the Whitehall Study, the Paris Prospective Study, and the Helsinki Policemen Study evaluated the relationship between hyperglycemia and mortality among non-diabetic men[59]. Men with fasting glucose levels in the upper 2.5% of values and upper 20% of 2-hour glucose levels after an oral glucose tolerance test demonstrated a significant increase in all-cause mortality when compared with those in lower distributions[55]. Men in the upper 2.5% of values for both fasting and 2-hour glucose levels were also at higher risk for cardiovascular and coronary artery disease-related death[59]. The Framingham Offspring Study investigated the effect of impaired glucose tolerance, impaired fasting glucose, and type 2 diabetes mellitus on the

development of coronary artery disease among patients without known cardiovascular disease[56]. Compared with those with normal glucose tolerance, patients with impaired glucose tolerance and impaired fasting glucose had a trend toward an increased incidence of subclinical coronary atherosclerosis as suggested by electron beam computed tomography (EBCT)[60]. Patients with overt diabetes were significantly more likely to have EBCT evidence of coronary artery disease[60]. Furthermore, patients with evidence of insulin resistance were twice as likely to have subclinical coronary atherosclerosis compared with those who did not[60]. The recent Strong Heart Study evaluated the relationship between prehypertension, impaired glucose tolerance, impaired fasting glucose, diabetes, and cardiovascular risk[16]. Compared with normotensive patients, patients with prehypertension only, prehypertension and impaired glucose tolerance, prehypertension and impaired fasting glucose, prehypertension and diabetes, and diabetes only had a significantly higher incidence of cardiovascular disease (Figure 7.17)[16].

The impact of overt diabetes and poor glycemic control on the risk of cardiovascular disease is well-established in the literature. Among patients with type

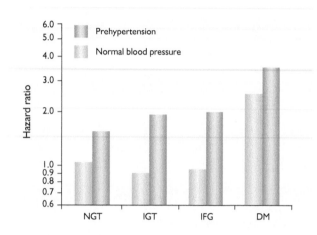

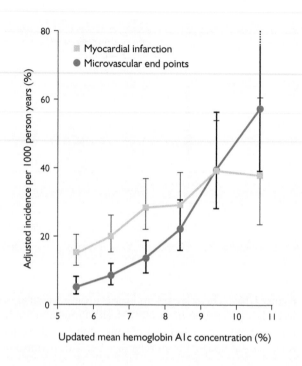

Figure 7.17 Hazard ratios for the incidence of cardiovascular disease associated with prehypertension and abnormalities of glucose metabolism. Hazard ratios were compared with the group of normal glucose tolerance and normal blood pressure and adjusted for age, gender, body mass index, waist circumference, low- and high-density lipoprotein cholesterol levels, triglycerides, physical activity, smoking, and alcohol use. NGT, normal glucose tolerance; IGT, impaired glucose tolerance; IFG, impaired fasting glucose; DM, diabetes mellitus. From reference 16, with permission

Figure 7.18 Incidence rates and 95% confidence intervals for myocardial infarction and microvascular complications plotted against mean hemoglobin A1c level. From reference 66, with permission

2 diabetes, one study demonstrated a significant increase in coronary artery disease-related death and coronary events associated with HbA1c levels of greater than 7.0% compared with lower levels[61]. The UKPDS 23 study evaluated a panel of proposed risk factors for coronary artery disease among patients with non-insulin dependent diabetes[62]. In addition to increased levels of LDL cholesterol, decreased levels of HDL cholesterol, hypertension, and smoking, hyperglycemia as determined by HbA1c levels was a significant predictor for the incidence of coronary artery disease[62]. Another study demonstrated that hyperglycemia as detected by HbA1c was also a strong predictor of stroke in patients with type 2 diabetes[63]. In the Munich General Practitioner Project, several risk predictors for macrovascular mortality were evaluated among patients with type 2 diabetes[64]. After 10 years of follow-up, HbA1c was demonstrated to be a significant risk predictor for macrovascular mortality[64]. Another study of diabetic patients including a large subset of Mexican-American patients

investigated the relationship of hyperglycemia to all-cause and cardiovascular mortality[65]. The study demonstrated that while diabetes was itself a strong predictor of all-cause and cardiovascular mortality, patients in the fourth quartile of baseline fasting plasma glucose experienced a 4.9-fold increase in all-cause mortality and a 4.7-fold increase in cardiovascular mortality[65]. The more recent UKPDS 35 study was designed to determine the relationship between hyperglycemia and the risk of macrovascular and microvascular complications in patients with type 2 diabetes[66]. The investigators found a significant relationship between increasing HbA1c level and the incidence of both macrovascular and microvascular disease (Figure 7.18)[66]. Furthermore, they found that each 1% reduction in mean HbA1c was associated with a 14% reduction in the risk of myocardial infarction[66]. In addition to hyperglycemia, microalbuminuria has also been shown to be a significant

(a)

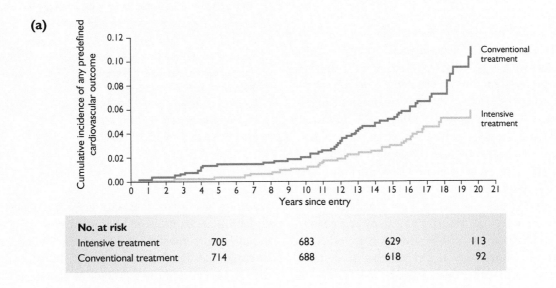

No. at risk				
Intensive treatment	705	683	629	113
Conventional treatment	714	688	618	92

(b)

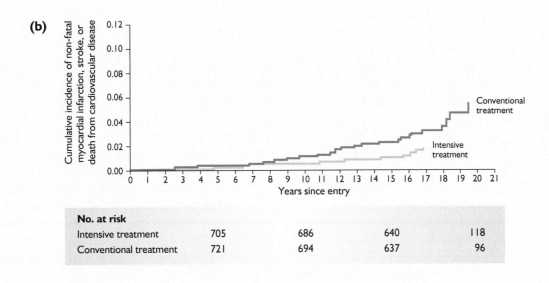

No. at risk				
Intensive treatment	705	686	640	118
Conventional treatment	721	694	637	96

Figure 7.19 Cumulative incidence of the first of any predefined cardiovascular disease outcome (a) and of the first occurrence of non-fatal myocardial infarction, stroke, or death from cardiovascular disease (b). From reference 72, with permission

independent predictor of coronary artery disease-related events in patients with diabetes[67].

Studies of patients with type 1 diabetes mellitus have also documented similar trends in cardiovascular disease and mortality. In a cohort study of 292 patients with juvenile-onset type 1 diabetes, the incidence of premature coronary artery disease was increased and the coronary artery disease-related mortality rate was markedly higher, especially among patients with renal complications, when compared with non-diabetic patients from the Framingham Heart Study[68]. The rates of angina, acute non-fatal myocardial infarction, and asymptomatic coronary artery disease as detected by stress test were also higher in type 1 diabetic patients[68]. The Diabetes UK cohort study followed 23 751 patients with type 1 diabetes to examine the difference in coronary artery disease-related mortality among diabetics and the general population[69]. At all ages, patients with type 1 diabetes had higher coronary artery disease-related mortality than the general population regardless of gender[69]. In the Pittsburgh insulin-dependent diabetes mellitus (IDDM) Morbidity and Mortality study, patients with type 1 diabetes older than 20 years of age were observed to have at least 20 times the mortality of the general US population[70]. A prospective study investigated the predictive value of several cardiovascular risk factors among patients with type 1 diabetes[71]. In multivariate Cox regression analysis, hyperglycemia as detected by high HbA1c levels was one of the only significant risk predictors after adjustment for other cardiovascular risk factors[71]. In the recent Diabetes Control and Complications Trial/ Epidemiology of Diabetes Interventions and Complications (DCCT/EDIC) Study, the effect of intensive glycemic control on the long-term incidence of cardiovascular disease was compared with that of standard therapy[72]. Intensive glycemic control led to significantly lower HbA1c levels and reduced the risk of any cardiovascular disease event by 42%, and the risk of non-fatal myocardial infarction, stroke, or death from cardiovascular disease by 57% compared with standard insulin therapy (Figure 7.19)[72]. These data suggest that hyperglycemia is associated with a significant increase in the risk of cardiovascular events and that intensive diabetes control is effective in mitigating this risk[72].

Based on the large number of studies linking disorders of glucose metabolism to the incidence of cardiovascular disease, the assessment of cardiometabolic risk factors should include consideration not only for overt diabetes mellitus, but also for other disorders on the spectrum such as impaired glucose tolerance, impaired fasting glucose, and insulin resistance.

THE METABOLIC SYNDROME

The metabolic syndrome is a recently defined constellation of known risk factors that has been associated with an increased risk of cardiovascular disease as well as the development of diabetes. While many of the cardiometabolic risk factors have the tendency to cluster in patients, the components of the metabolic

Table 7.5 NCEP ATP III criteria for the metabolic syndrome. From reference 33, with permission

Increased waist circumference (in men > 40 inches (> 102 cm) and in women > 35 inches (> 88 cm))
Elevated triglycerides (≥ 150 mg/dL)
Low HDL cholesterol (men < 40 mg/dL and women < 50 mg/dL)
High blood pressure (≥ 130/85 mmHg)
Impaired fasting glucose (≥ 110 mg/dL)

syndrome occur together with great frequency. Several definitions of the metabolic syndrome exist including ones from the NCEP ATP III, the WHO, and the International Diabetes Federation. In general, most definitions endorse the following basic criteria: a measure of abdominal adiposity, hypertriglyceridemia, low HDL cholesterol levels, hypertension, and evidence of impaired glucose metabolism. The NCEP ATP III defines the metabolic syndrome as any three of the following: elevated triglycerides (≥ 150 mg/dL), low HDL cholesterol (men < 40 mg/dL and women < 50 mg/dL), impaired fasting glucose (≥ 110 mg/dL), high blood pressure (≥ 130/85 mmHg), and increased waist circumference (men > 40 inches, or > 102 cm, and women > 35 inches, or > 88 cm) (Table 7.5)[33]. The prevalence of the metabolic syndrome has steadily increased especially among middle-aged adults in the US, in part because of increasing clinician comfort with diagnosis, but also secondary to increasing prevalence of risk factors such as abdominal obesity[73]. The unadjusted prevalence of the metabolic syndrome was 23.1% among participants in NHANES III (1988–1994) compared with 26.7% in NHANES 1999–2000[73].

Numerous studies have established the metabolic syndrome as an important marker of cardiovascular risk. In a study of 4483 patients, the relationship between the metabolic syndrome as defined by the WHO criteria (which include microalbuminuria in place of impaired fasting glucose) and cardiovascular risk was examined[74]. Patients meeting criteria for the metabolic syndrome experienced a 3-fold increase in the risk of coronary artery disease and stroke[74]. Cardiovascular mortality was increased to 12% among patients with the metabolic syndrome compared with 2.2% in patients not meeting the WHO definition[74]. Of the various criteria constituting the WHO

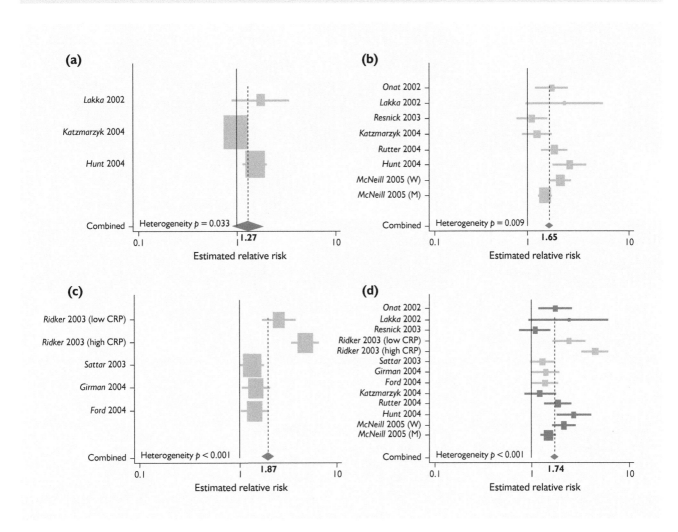

Figure 7.20 Associations between the metabolic syndrome, using the National Cholesterol Education Program (NCEP) definition, and all-cause mortality (a); associations between the metabolic syndrome, using the NCEP definition, and cardiovascular disease (b); associations between the metabolic syndrome, using a modified NCEP definition, and cardiovascular disease (c); associations between the metabolic syndrome, using the NCEP and a modified NCEP definition, and cardiovascular disease (d). Blue, studies using the NCEP definition; yellow, studies using a modified NCEP definition; M, men; W, women; CRP, C-reactive protein. From reference 76, with permission

definition, microalbuminuria conferred the greatest risk of cardiovascular mortality with a relative risk increase of 2.8[74]. In a cohort study of patients participating in the Framingham Heart Study, the risk of cardiovascular disease and coronary artery disease was evaluated in patients with the metabolic syndrome[75]. For men, the metabolic syndrome age-adjusted relative risk was 2.88 (95% CI 1.99–4.16) for cardiovascular disease and 2.54 (95% CI 1.62–3.98) for coronary artery disease[75]. Among women, the metabolic syndrome was associated with a relative risk of 2.25 (95% CI 1.31–3.88) for cardiovascular disease and 1.54 (95%

CI 0.68–3.53) for coronary artery disease[75]. Recently, an analysis of several prospective studies evaluated the impact of the metabolic syndrome on the relative risk of all-cause mortality and cardiovascular disease (Figure 7.20)[76]. For studies using the exact NCEP definition, the metabolic syndrome was associated with a relative risk of 1.27 (95% CI 0.90–1.78) for all-cause mortality and 1.65 (95% CI 1.38–1.99) for cardiovascular disease[76]. Among studies using the exact WHO definition, the metabolic syndrome was associated with a relative risk of 1.37 (95% CI 1.09–1.74) for all-cause mortality, 1.93 (95% CI 1.39–2.67) for cardiovascular

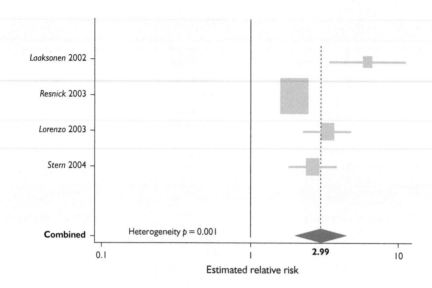

Figure 7.21 Associations between the metabolic syndrome, using the NCEP definition, and diabetes. From reference 76, with permission

disease, and 2.60 (95% CI 1.55–4.38) for coronary artery disease[76]. Regardless of the definition utilized to diagnose it, the weight of evidence from these studies supports the metabolic syndrome as an important risk factor for cardiovascular events.

In addition to its role as a risk factor for cardiovascular disease, the metabolic syndrome is also an important predictor for the development of diabetes. In an analysis of patients enrolled in the Framingham Heart Study, the metabolic syndrome was associated with significant relative risks for the development of type 2 diabetes of 6.92 in men and 6.90 in women[75]. A recent analysis of prospective studies using the NCEP and WHO definitions evaluated the relationship between the metabolic syndrome and the incidence of diabetes[76]. Patients meeting the NCEP definition of the metabolic syndrome demonstrated a significant relative risk of 2.99 (95% CI 1.96–4.57) for the development of diabetes (Figure 7.21)[76].

Comprised of known cardiovascular risk factors, the metabolic syndrome has emerged as an important independent disorder that places patients at an increased risk for both cardiovascular events and the development of type 2 diabetes. A comprehensive cardiometabolic assessment should include screening for this group of risk factors.

SMOKING

Smoking remains one of the most potent modifiable risk factors for cardiovascular disease. Despite numerous studies documenting the cardiovascular sequelae of smoking and multiple public education campaigns, a significant subset of the US population continues to smoke. Smokers not only place themselves at risk for cardiovascular events, but also those around them as increasing data suggest that second-hand smoke is an underestimated and under-recognized risk factor.

Smoking is a significant and independent risk factor for coronary artery disease, stroke, peripheral vascular disease, and increased cardiovascular mortality. A prospective cohort study performed in South Korea evaluated the effect of cigarette smoking on the incidence of cardiovascular disease among men with relatively low serum total cholesterol levels[77]. Smoking was found to be a significant independent risk factor for coronary artery disease, cerebrovascular disease, and total atherosclerotic cardiovascular disease[77]. In the Finnmark Study, the incidence of myocardial infarction was increased 6-fold in women and 3-fold in men who smoked at least 20 cigarettes a day compared with patients who had never smoked[78]. The Finnmark Study suggested that women may be more susceptible to the cardiovascular effects of smoking when compared with men[78]. In a subsequent study, female smokers demonstrated a relative risk for myocardial infarction of 2.24 compared with a relative risk of 1.43 among male smokers[79]. This gender difference did not attenuate even after adjustment for other major cardiovascular risk factors such as hypertension, total and HDL cholesterol, triglyceride levels, and diabetes[79]. The INTERHEART study evaluated the contributions of several known cardiovascular risk factors including smoking to the incidence of myocardial infarction among patients from 52 countries and every inhabited continent[25]. Among several other risk factors, smoking was shown to be a significant contributor to the risk of developing acute myocardial infarction among this 'real world' patient population[25]. A cohort study of Finnish men investigated the relationship between cigarette smoking and all-cause and coronary artery disease-related mortality[80]. At 35 years of follow-up, persistent smoking correlated with a significant increase in all-cause and coronary artery disease-related mortality[80]. Smoking is also associated with adverse outcomes among patients with established cardiovascular disease. In a follow-up study from the Bezafibrate Infarction Prevention (BIP) trial, smoking was found to be a potent independent risk predictor for sudden cardiac death among patients with known coronary artery disease[81]. Among patients who have undergone percutaneous coronary revascularization, persistent smoking has been shown to increase significantly the risk of death and Q-wave myocardial infarction[82]. Among patients with left ventricular systolic dysfunction in the SOLVD trial, persistent smoking was associated with significant increases in all-cause mortality and the incidence of death, recurrent congestive heart failure requiring hospital admission, or myocardial infarction[83].

Several studies have also established passive smoking, or second-hand smoke, as a significant cardiovascular risk factor. The Nurses' Health Study assessed exposure to passive smoking at home and at work, and its relationship to the incidence of coronary artery disease in non-smoking women[84]. Non-smoking women exposed to second-hand smoke demonstrated almost twice the incidence of coronary artery disease as compared with women not exposed to environmental smoke[84]. A large meta-analysis evaluated 18 epidemiological studies to define the risk of coronary artery disease associated with passive smoking[85]. The study revealed that both male and female non-smokers exposed to passive smoking experienced approximately a 25% increase in the relative risk of coronary artery disease and that the increased risk followed a dose–response relationship[85]. In the American Cancer Society's Cancer Prevention Study II, a cohort of 353 180 women and 126 500 men was followed to assess the relationship between self-reported passive exposure to tobacco smoke and the incidence of coronary artery disease[86]. After adjustment for other major cardiovascular risk factors, non-smoking patients exposed to second-hand smoke demonstrated an approximately 20% higher rate of death from coronary artery disease than those not exposed to environmental smoke[86]. A recent review has shown that the large majority of epidemiological studies have established second-hand smoke as a significant risk factor for coronary artery disease (Figure 7.22)[87].

Based on the data presented above, both active and passive smoking should be considered as potent and modifiable cardiovascular risk factors. A complete cardiometabolic risk assessment should include screening for smoking as well as exposure to second-hand smoke.

INFLAMMATORY MARKERS

An improved understanding of the pathophysiology of atherosclerosis and atherothrombosis has given rise to an increasing interest in the role of inflammation in the pathogenesis of cardiovascular disease. Chronic inflammation, including a strong macrophage response triggered by vascular injury, oxidized LDL cholesterol, and possibly infection, drives the process of atherosclerosis leading to the development of vulnerable plaques[88] (Figure 7.23). Rupture of these vulnerable atherosclerotic plaques leads to an acute inflammatory response that gives rise to the process of atherothrombosis and ultimately ACS[88]. A growing body of evidence has suggested that elevated markers of systemic inflammation, such as C-reactive protein (CRP), interleukin 6 (IL-6), serum amyloid A (SAA), and tumor necrosis factor α, are important predictors of cardiovascular risk. CRP remains the most important of these markers of inflammation as the majority of studies have validated CRP as the most potent and consistent predictor of cardiovascular risk (Figure 7.24). Furthermore, CRP is currently the best studied

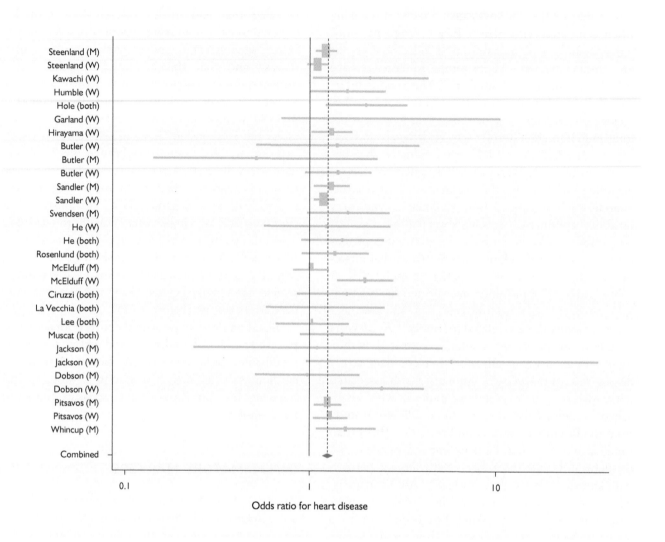

Figure 7.22   Summary of epidemiological studies on the relationship between passive smoking and the incidence of coronary artery disease and the results of random-effects meta-analysis. M, men; W, women. From reference 87, with permission

systemic marker of inflammation that is widely available means of detection.

Numerous studies have validated CRP as a marker of systemic inflammation and as a strong predictor of cardiovascular disease. A study of men in the Honolulu Heart Program was designed to evaluate the relationship between CRP and the incidence of myocardial infarction[91]. After adjustment for major cardiovascular risk factors, the odds of myocardial infarction increased with progressive elevation in CRP[91]. A prospective case–control analysis of patients enrolled in the Physicians' Health Study investigated the value of CRP as a risk predictor for sudden cardiac death[92].

Patients in the highest quartile of CRP demonstrated a 2.78-fold increase in the risk of sudden cardiac death when compared with the lowest quartile[92]. The significance of CRP as a risk predictor of sudden cardiac death persisted even after adjustment for other cardiovascular risk factors[92]. In an analysis of patients enrolled in the Cholesterol and Recurrent Events (CARE) trial, CRP and SAA levels from post-myocardial infarction patients who experienced recurrent non-fatal myocardial infarction or a fatal coronary event were compared with levels from patients who remained free from recurrent events[93]. Patients with a CRP level within the highest quintile experienced a

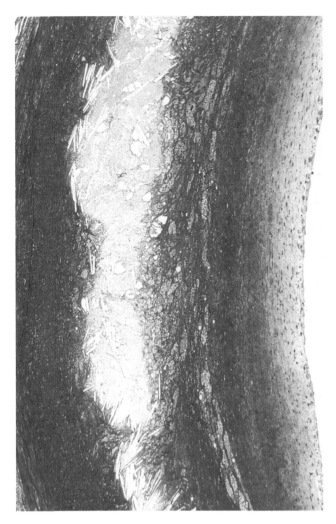

Figure 7.23 Atheroma at the left main coronary artery bifurcation. Extracellular lipid, including cholesterol crystals, makes up the lipid core. In addition to causing thickening of the arterial wall, the accumulated lipid may weaken the wall by displacing the structual smooth muscle cells that are normally present at this location. From Stary HC. Atlas of Atherosclerosis: Progression and Regression, 2nd edn. Lancaster, UK: Parthenon Publishing, 2003: 78 (reference 89), with permission

75% increase in the relative risk of recurrent events when compared with patients with values in the lowest quintile (Figure 7.25)[93]. A similar trend was observed for SAA levels[93]. In an analysis of patients participating in the Physicians' Health Study, men with baseline plasma CRP levels within the highest quartile were approximately three times as likely to experience myocardial infarction and almost twice as likely to suffer from an ischemic stroke when com-

pared with patients with values in the lowest quartile[94]. These trends persisted even after adjustment for smoking and lipid-related and non-lipid-related risk factors[94]. Among patients enrolled in the Women's Health Initiative, baseline CRP and IL-6 levels were both significantly associated with a 2-fold increase in the odds of a coronary artery disease-related event after adjustment for lipid and non-lipid risk factors[95]. Among the various systemic markers evaluated including SAA and IL-6, CRP appears to be the strongest and most consistent predictor of cardiovascular risk (Figure 7.26)[96]. A recent analysis of patients enrolled in the Women's Health Study investigated the relationship between CRP, LDL cholesterol, and the incidence of cardiovascular events[97]. After adjustment for age, smoking status, diabetes, hypertension, and use of hormone replacement therapy, higher quintiles of both CRP and LDL cholesterol were significantly associated with an increasing relative risk for cardiovascular events[97]. However, CRP proved to be a stronger predictor of cardiovascular events than LDL cholesterol[97]. In addition, 77% of events occurred in patients with LDL cholesterol levels of less than 160 mg/dL and 46% of events occurred in those with LDL cholesterol levels below 130 mg/dL[97]. These data suggest that CRP identified patients who remained at high risk for cardiovascular events despite favorable LDL cholesterol levels[97]. Furthermore, this study demonstrated that CRP adds additional prognostic information to both LDL cholesterol and the Framingham Risk Score (Figure 7.27)[97].

In addition to its role in cardiovascular disease, inflammation is also believed to play a significant role in the pathogenesis of diabetes. In a prospective case–control study of healthy middle-aged patients enrolled in the Women's Health Study, the relationship between the incidence of type 2 diabetes and the inflammatory markers CRP and IL-6 was investigated[98]. The incidence of confirmed clinically diagnosed type 2 diabetes was significantly more common among patients with elevated levels of CRP and IL-6[98]. The relative risk for developing diabetes among women in the highest quartile of inflammatory marker levels compared with the lowest quartile was 15.7 for CRP and 7.5 for IL-6[98]. A significant positive relationship between inflammatory markers and the incidence of diabetes persisted even after adjustment for BMI, family history of diabetes, smoking, exercise, use of alcohol, and hormone replacement therapy[98]. The results

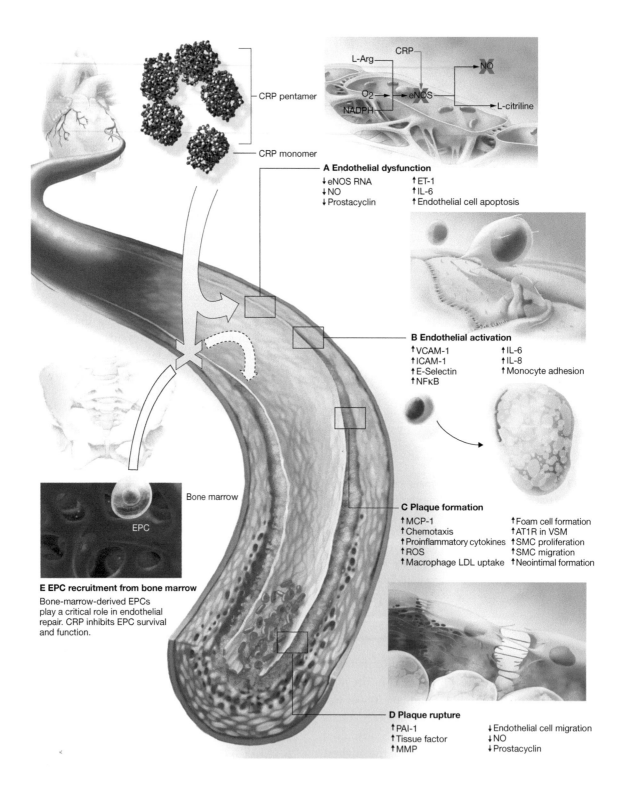

A Endothelial dysfunction

↓eNOS RNA	↑ET-1
↓NO	↑IL-6
↓Prostacyclin	↑Endothelial cell apoptosis

B Endothelial activation

↑VCAM-1	↑IL-6
↑ICAM-1	↑IL-8
↑E-Selectin	↑Monocyte adhesion
↑NFκB	

C Plaque formation

↑MCP-1	↑Foam cell formation
↑Chemotaxis	↑AT1R in VSM
↑Proinflammatory cytokines	↑SMC proliferation
↑ROS	↑SMC migration
↑Macrophage LDL uptake	↑Neointimal formation

E EPC recruitment from bone marrow

Bone-marrow-derived EPCs play a critical role in endothelial repair. CRP inhibits EPC survival and function.

D Plaque rupture

↑PAI-1	↓Endothelial cell migration
↑Tissue factor	↓NO
↑MMP	↓Prostacyclin

Figure 7.24 CRP participates in key processes linked to atherothrombosis. Reprinted from reference 90, with permission

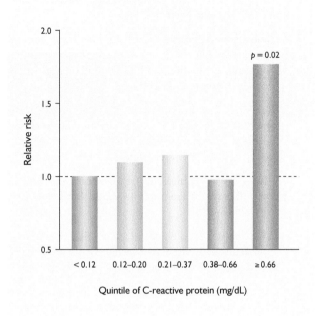

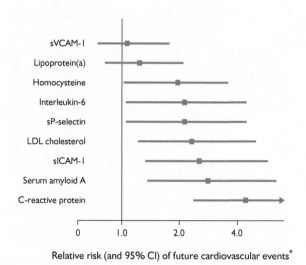

Figure 7.25 Relative risk of recurrent events among post-myocardial infarction patients according to baseline plasma concentration of C-reactive protein. From reference 93, with permission

Figure 7.26 Prognostic value of various cardiovascular and inflammatory biomarkers in healthy women enrolled in the Women's Health Study. *Top vs. bottom quartile after adjustment for age and smoking; sVCAM-1, soluble vascular adhesion molecule-1; sICAM-1, soluble intracellular adhesion molecule-1. From reference 96, with permission

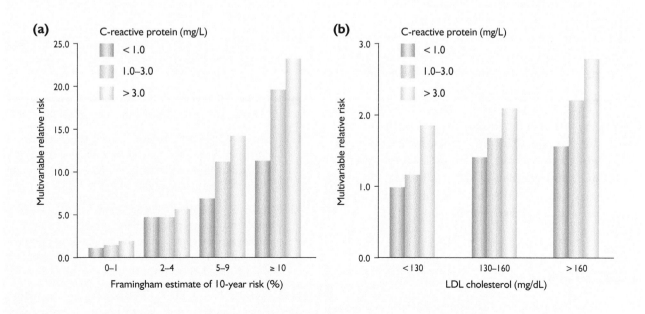

Figure 7.27 Multivariable-adjusted relative risks of cardiovascular disease according to levels of CRP and the estimated 10-year risk based on the Framingham Risk Score as defined by the National Cholesterol Education Program (a), and according to levels of CRP and categories of LDL cholesterol (b). From reference 97, with permission

of this study support the hypothesis that inflammation may play a significant role in the pathogenesis of type 2 diabetes and that markers of inflammation such as CRP may be important risk predictors for diabetes.

While the most effective way to utilize measures of systemic inflammation in cardiovascular risk assessment is still being evaluated, a significant body of evidence suggests that these markers are important predictors of cardiovascular events. Markers of systemic inflammation appear to be independent predictors of cardiovascular risk and may help to identify high-risk patients who would not be recognized as such using conventional risk factors such as LDL cholesterol. Of these markers of systemic inflammation, CRP offers the greatest opportunity for clinical utility given that it has a widely available assay and a strong correlation with cardiovascular risk.

CONCLUSIONS

The importance of the concept of assessing overall cardiometabolic risk is highlighted by the fact that cardiovascular risk factors do not occur in isolation of each other and that some predispose patients to other risk factors. The majority of patients present with multiple cardiometabolic risk factors, and their cardiovascular outcomes are driven by combinations of these risk factors which are often more potent than suggested by their sums. Cardiometabolic risk encompasses emerging risk predictors, such as the metabolic syndrome and markers of inflammation, that may be present in patients without other more traditional risk factors. An evaluation that only assesses for traditional risk factors may fail to identify patients at elevated risk for adverse cardiovascular outcomes. Therefore, assessment and knowledge of all the cardiometabolic risk factors and associated risks have become a crucial part of cardiovascular risk assessment.

REFERENCES

1. Hajjar I, Kotchen TA. Trends in prevalence, awareness, treatment, and control of hypertension in the United States, 1988–2000. JAMA 2003; 290: 199–206

2. World Health Organization. World Health Report 2002: Reducing risks, promoting healthy life. Geneva, Switzerland: World Health Organization, 2002. http://www.who.int/whr/2002

3. Chobanian AV, Bakris GL, Black HR, et al. Seventh report of the Joint National Committee on Prevention, Detection, Evaluation, and Treatment of High Blood Pressure. Hypertension 2003; 42: 1206–52

4. Burt VL, Whelton P, Roccella EJ, et al. Prevalence of hypertension in the US adult population. Results from the Third National Health and Nutrition Examination Survey, 1988–1991. Hypertension 1995; 25: 305–13

5. Wilson PW. Established risk factors and coronary artery disease: the Framingham Study. Am J Hypertens 1994; 7: 7S–12S

6. Lloyd-Jones DM, Leip EP, Larson MG, et al. Novel approach to examining first cardiovascular events after hypertension onset. Hypertension 2005; 45: 39–45

7. Lloyd-Jones DM, Evans JC, Levy D. Hypertension in adults across the age spectrum: current outcomes and control in the community. JAMA 2005; 294: 466–72

8. Pastor-Barriuso R, Banegas JR, Damian J, et al. Systolic blood pressure, diastolic blood pressure, and pulse pressure: an evaluation of their joint effect on mortality. Ann Intern Med 2003; 139: 731–9

9. Lewington S, Clarke R, Qizilbash N, et al. Age-specific relevance of usual blood pressure to vascular mortality: a meta-analysis of individual data for one million adults in 61 prospective studies. Lancet 2002; 360: 1903–13

10. Vasan RS, Larson MG, Leip EP, et al. Impact of high-normal blood pressure on the risk of cardiovascular disease. N Engl J Med 2001; 345: 1291–7

11. Semple PF, Lindop GBM. An Atlas of Hypertension, 2nd edn. Lancaster, UK: Parthenon Publishing, 1998

12. Gress TW, Nieto FJ, Shahar E, et al. Hypertension and antihypertensive therapy as risk factors for type 2 diabetes mellitus. Atherosclerosis Risk in Communities Study. N Engl J Med 2000; 342: 905–12

13. Yusuf S, Sleight P, Pogue J, et al. Effects of an angiotensin-converting-enzyme inhibitor, ramipril, on cardiovascular events in high-risk patients. The Heart Outcomes Prevention Evaluation Study Investigators. N Engl J Med 2000; 342: 145–53

14. Curb JD, Pressel SL, Cutler JA, et al. Effect of diuretic-based antihypertensive treatment on cardiovascular disease risk in older diabetic patients with isolated systolic hypertension. Systolic Hypertension in the Elderly Program Cooperative Research Group. JAMA 1996; 276: 1886–92

15. Tuomilehto J, Rastenyte D, Birkenhager WH, et al. Effects of calcium-channel blockade in older patients with diabetes and systolic hypertension. Systolic Hypertension in Europe Trial Investigators. N Engl J Med 1999; 340: 677–84

16. Zhang Y, Lee ET, Devereux RB, et al. Prehypertension, diabetes, and cardiovascular disease risk in a population-based sample: the Strong Heart Study. Hypertension 2006; 47: 410–14

17. World Health Organization. Global strategy on diet, physical activity and health. Geneva, Switzerland: World Health Organization 2006. Available at: http://www.who.int/dietphysicalactivity/media/en/gsfs_obesity.pdf

18. Pouliot MC, Despres JP, Lemieux S, et al. Waist circumference and abdominal sagittal diameter: best simple anthropometric indexes of abdominal visceral adipose tissue accumulation and related cardiovascular risk in men and women. Am J Cardiol 1994; 73: 460–8

19. Ford ES, Mokdad AH, Giles WH. Trends in waist circumference among US adults. Obes Res 2003; 11: 1223–31

20. Calle EE, Thun MJ, Petrelli JM, et al. Body-mass index and mortality in a prospective cohort of US adults. N Engl J Med 1999; 341: 1097–105

21. Wilson PW, Kannel WB, Silbershatz H, D'Agostino RB. Clustering of metabolic factors and coronary heart disease. Arch Intern Med 1999; 159: 1104–9

22. Peeters A, Barendregt JJ, Willekens F, et al. Obesity in adulthood and its consequences for life expectancy: a life-table analysis. Ann Intern Med 2003; 138: 24–32

23. Dagenais GR, Yi Q, Mann JF, et al. Prognostic impact of body weight and abdominal obesity in women and men with cardiovascular disease. Am Heart J 2005; 149: 54–60

24. Lyon CJ, Law RE, Hsueh WA. Minireview: adiposity, inflammation, and atherogenesis. Endocrinology 2003; 144: 2195–200

25. Yusuf S, Hawken S, Ounpuu S, et al. Effect of potentially modifiable risk factors associated with myocardial infarction in 52 countries (the INTERHEART study): case-control study. Lancet 2004; 364: 937–52

26. Rexrode KM, Carey VJ, Hennekens CH, et al. Abdominal adiposity and coronary heart disease in women. JAMA 1998; 280: 1843–8

27. Empana JP, Ducimetiere P, Charles MA, Jouven X. Sagittal abdominal diameter and risk of sudden death in asymptomatic middle-aged men: the Paris Prospective Study I. Circulation 2004; 110: 2781–5

28. Zraika S, Dunlop M, Proietto J, Andrikopoulos S. Effects of free fatty acids on insulin secretion in obesity. Obes Rev 2002; 3: 103–12

29. Banerji MA, Faridi N, Atluri R, et al. Body composition, visceral fat, leptin, and insulin resistance in Asian Indian men. J Clin Endocrinol Metab 1999; 84: 137–44

30. Wang Y, Rimm EB, Stampfer MJ, et al. Comparison of abdominal adiposity and overall obesity in predicting risk of type 2 diabetes among men. Am J Clin Nutr 2005; 81: 555–63

31. Knowler WC, Barrett-Connor E, Fowler SE, et al. Reduction in the incidence of type 2 diabetes with lifestyle intervention or metformin. N Engl J Med 2002; 346: 393–403

32. Genest J Jr, McNamara JR, Ordovas JM, et al. Lipoprotein cholesterol, apolipoprotein A-I and B and lipoprotein (a) abnormalities in men with premature coronary artery disease. J Am Coll Cardiol 1992; 19: 792–802

33. National Cholesterol Education Program (NCEP) Expert Panel on Detection, Evaluation, and Treatment of High Blood Cholesterol in Adults (Adult Treatment Panel III). Third Report of the National Cholesterol Education Program (NCEP) Expert Panel on Detection, Evaluation and Treatment of High Blood Cholesterol in Adults (Adult Treatment Panel III) final report. Circulation 2002; 106: 3143–421

34. Castelli WP. Cholesterol and lipids in the risk of coronary artery disease – the Framingham Heart Study. Can J Cardiol 1988; 4 (Suppl A): 5A–10A

35. Castelli WP, Garrison RJ, Wilson PW, et al. Incidence of coronary heart disease and lipoprotein cholesterol levels. The Framingham Study. JAMA 1986; 256: 2835–8

36. Stampfer MJ, Sacks FM, Salvini S, et al. A prospective study of cholesterol, apolipoproteins, and the risk of myocardial infarction. N Engl J Med 1991; 325: 373–81

37. Weverling-Rijnsburger AW, Jonkers IJ, van Exel E, et al. High-density vs low-density lipoprotein cholesterol as the risk factor for coronary artery disease and stroke in old age. Arch Intern Med 2003; 163: 1549–54

38. Shah PK, Amin J. Low high density lipoprotein level is associated with increased restenosis rate after coronary angioplasty. Circulation 1992; 85: 1279–85

39. Pearson TA, Bulkley BH, Achuff SC, et al. The association of low levels of HDL cholesterol and arteriographically defined coronary artery disease. Am J Epidemiol 1979; 109: 285–95

40. Miller M, Seidler A, Kwiterovich PO, Pearson TA. Long-term predictors of subsequent cardiovascular events with coronary artery disease and 'desirable' levels of plasma total cholesterol. Circulation 1992; 86: 1165–70

41. Nissen SE, Tuzcu EM, Schoenhagen P, et al. Effect of intensive compared with moderate lipid-lowering therapy on progression of coronary atherosclerosis: a randomized controlled trial. JAMA 2004; 291: 1071–80

42. Pekkanen J, Linn S, Heiss G, et al. Ten-year mortality from cardiovascular disease in relation to cholesterol level among men with and without preexisting cardiovascular disease. N Engl J Med 1990; 322: 1700–7

43. Wilson PW, D'Agostino RB, Levy D, et al. Prediction of coronary heart disease using risk factor categories. Circulation 1998; 97: 1837–47

44. The Lipid Research Clinics Coronary Primary Prevention Trial results. I. Reduction in incidence of coronary heart disease. JAMA 1984; 251: 351–64

45. The Lipid Research Clinics Coronary Primary Prevention Trial results. II. The relationship of reduction in incidence of coronary heart disease to cholesterol lowering. JAMA 1984; 251: 365–74

46. Shepherd J, Cobbe SM, Ford I, et al. Prevention of coronary heart disease with pravastatin in men with hypercholesterolemia. West of Scotland Coronary Prevention Study Group. N Engl J Med 1995; 333: 1301–7

47. Downs JR, Clearfield M, Weis S, et al. Primary prevention of acute coronary events with lovastatin in men and women with average cholesterol levels: results of AFCAPS/TexCAPS. Air Force/Texas Coronary Atherosclerosis Prevention Study. JAMA 1998; 279: 1615–22

48. Falk E. Pathogenesis of atherosclerosis. J Am Coll Cardiol 2006; 47 (Suppl C): C7–12

49. Wilensky RL, Hee Kwon Song, Ferrari VA. Role of magnetic resonance and intravascular magnetic resonance in the detection of vulnerable plaques. Am Coll Cardiol, 2006; 47 (Suppl C): C48–56

50. Sacks FM, Pfeffer MA, Moye LA, et al. The effect of pravastatin on coronary events after myocardial infarction in patients with average cholesterol levels. Cholesterol and Recurrent Events Trial investigators. N Engl J Med 1996; 335: 1001–9

51. Heart Protection Study Collaborative Group. MRC/BHF Heart Protection Study of cholesterol lowering with simvastatin in 20 536 high-risk individuals: a randomised placebo-controlled trial. Lancet 2002; 360: 7–22

52. Cannon CP, Braunwald E, McCabe CH, et al. Intensive versus moderate lipid lowering with statins after acute coronary syndromes. N Engl J Med 2004; 350: 1495–504

53. de Lemos JA, Blazing MA, Wiviott SD, et al. Early intensive vs a delayed conservative simvastatin strategy in patients with acute coronary syndromes: phase Z of the A to Z trial. JAMA 2004; 292: 1307–16

54. LaRosa JC, Grundy SM, Waters DD, et al. Intensive lipid lowering with atorvastatin in patients with stable coronary disease. N Engl J Med 2005; 352: 1425–35

55. Pedersen TR, Faergeman O, Kastelein JJ, et al. High-dose atorvastatin vs usual-dose simvastatin for secondary prevention after myocardial infarction: the IDEAL study: a randomized controlled trial. JAMA 2005; 294: 2437–45

56. Hokanson JE, Austin MA. Plasma triglyceride level is a risk factor for cardiovascular disease independent of high-density lipoprotein cholesterol level: a meta-analysis of population-based prospective studies. J Cardiovasc Risk 1996; 3: 213–19

57. Assmann G, Schulte H, von Eckardstein A. Hypertriglyceridemia and elevated lipoprotein(a) are risk factors for major coronary events in middle-aged men. Am J Cardiol 1996; 77: 1179–84

58. Yarnell JW, Patterson CC, Sweetnam PM, et al. Do total and high density lipoprotein cholesterol and triglycerides act independently in the prediction of ischemic heart disease? Ten-year follow-up of Caerphilly and Speedwell Cohorts. Arterioscler Thromb Vasc Biol 2001; 21: 1340–5

59. Balkau B, Shipley M, Jarrett RJ, et al. High blood glucose concentration is a risk factor for mortality in middle-aged nondiabetic men. 20-year follow-up in the Whitehall Study, the Paris Prospective Study, and the Helsinki Policemen Study. Diabetes Care 1998; 21: 360–7

60. Meigs JB, Larson MG, D'Agostino RB, et al. Coronary artery calcification in type 2 diabetes and insulin resistance: the Framingham Offspring Study. Diabetes Care 2002; 25: 1313–19

61. Kuusisto J, Mykkanen L, Pyorala K, Laakso M. NIDDM and its metabolic control predict coronary heart disease in elderly subjects. Diabetes 1994; 43: 960–7

62. Turner RC, Millns H, Neil HA, et al. Risk factors for coronary artery disease in non-insulin dependent diabetes mellitus: United Kingdom Prospective Diabetes Study (UKPDS: 23). Br Med J 1998; 316: 823–8

63. Lehto S, Ronnemaa T, Pyorala K, Laakso M. Predictors of stroke in middle-aged patients with non-insulin-dependent diabetes. Stroke 1996; 27: 63–8

64. Standl E, Balletshofer B, Dahl B, et al. Predictors of 10-year macrovascular and overall mortality in patients with NIDDM: the Munich General Practitioner Project. Diabetologia 1996; 39: 1540–5

65. Wei M, Gaskill SP, Haffner SM, Stern MP. Effects of diabetes and level of glycemia on all-cause and cardiovascular mortality. The San Antonio Heart Study. Diabetes Care 1998; 21: 1167–72

66. Stratton IM, Adler AI, Neil HA, et al. Association of glycaemia with macrovascular and microvascular complications of type 2 diabetes (UKPDS 35): prospective observational study. Br Med J 2000; 321: 405–12

67. Rutter MK, Wahid ST, McComb JM, Marshall SM. Significance of silent ischemia and microalbuminuria in predicting coronary events in asymptomatic patients with type 2 diabetes. J Am Coll Cardiol 2002; 40: 56–61

68. Krolewski AS, Kosinski EJ, Warram JH, et al. Magnitude and determinants of coronary artery disease in juvenile-onset, insulin-dependent diabetes mellitus. Am J Cardiol 1987; 59: 750–5

69. Laing SP, Swerdlow AJ, Slater SD, et al. Mortality from heart disease in a cohort of 23,000 patients with insulin-treated diabetes. Diabetologia 2003; 46: 760–5

70. Dorman JS, Laporte RE, Kuller LH, et al. The Pittsburgh insulin-dependent diabetes mellitus (IDDM) morbidity and mortality study. Mortality results. Diabetes 1984; 33: 271–6

71. Lehto S, Ronnemaa T, Pyorala K, Laakso M. Poor glycemic control predicts coronary heart disease events in patients with type 1 diabetes without nephropathy. Arterioscler Thromb Vasc Biol 1999; 19: 1014–19

72. Nathan DM, Cleary PA, Backlund JY, et al. Intensive diabetes treatment and cardiovascular disease in patients with type 1 diabetes. N Engl J Med 2005; 353: 2643–53

73. Ford ES, Giles WH, Mokdad AH. Increasing prevalence of the metabolic syndrome among US Adults. Diabetes Care 2004; 27: 2444–9

74. Isomaa B, Almgren P, Tuomi T, et al. Cardiovascular morbidity and mortality associated with the metabolic syndrome. Diabetes Care 2001; 24: 683–9

75. Wilson PW, D'Agostino RB, Parise H, et al. Metabolic syndrome as a precursor of cardiovascular disease and type 2 diabetes mellitus. Circulation 2005; 112: 3066–72

76. Ford ES. Risks for all-cause mortality, cardiovascular disease, and diabetes associated with the metabolic syndrome: a summary of the evidence. Diabetes Care 2005; 28: 1769–78

77. Jee SH, Suh I, Kim IS, Appel LJ. Smoking and atherosclerotic cardiovascular disease in men with low levels of serum cholesterol: the Korea Medical Insurance Corporation Study. JAMA 1999; 282: 2149–55

78. Njolstad I, Arnesen E, Lund-Larsen PG. Smoking, serum lipids, blood pressure, and sex differences in myocardial infarction. A 12-year follow-up of the Finnmark Study. Circulation 1996; 93: 450–6

79. Prescott E, Hippe M, Schnohr P, et al. Smoking and risk of myocardial infarction in women and men: longitudinal population study. Br Med J 1998; 316: 1043–7

80. Qiao Q, Tervahauta M, Nissinen A, Tuomilehto J. Mortality from all causes and from coronary heart disease related to smoking and changes in smoking during a 35-year follow-up of middle-aged Finnish men. Eur Heart J 2000; 21: 1621–6

81. Goldenberg I, Jonas M, Tenenbaum A, et al. Current smoking, smoking cessation, and the risk of sudden cardiac death in patients with coronary artery disease. Arch Intern Med 2003; 163: 2301–5

82. Hasdai D, Garratt KN, Grill DE, et al. Effect of smoking status on the long-term outcome after successful percutaneous coronary revascularization. N Engl J Med 1997; 336: 755–61

83. Suskin N, Sheth T, Negassa A, Yusuf S. Relationship of current and past smoking to mortality and morbidity in patients with left ventricular dysfunction. J Am Coll Cardiol 2001; 37: 1677–82

84. Kawachi I, Colditz GA, Speizer FE, et al. A prospective study of passive smoking and coronary heart disease. Circulation 1997; 95: 2374–9

85. He J, Vupputuri S, Allen K, et al. Passive smoking and the risk of coronary heart disease – a meta-analysis of epidemiologic studies. N Engl J Med 1999; 340: 920–6

86. Steenland K, Thun M, Lally C, Heath C Jr. Environmental tobacco smoke and coronary heart disease in the American Cancer Society CPS-II cohort. Circulation 1996; 94: 622–8

87. Barnoya J, Glantz SA. Cardiovascular effects of secondhand smoke: nearly as large as smoking. Circulation 2005; 111: 2684–98

88. Willerson JT, Ridker PM. Inflammation as a cardiovascular risk factor. Circulation 2004; 109 (Suppl 1): II2–10

89. Stary HC. Atlas of Atherosclerosis: Progression and Regression, 2nd edn. Lancaster: Parthenon Publishing, 2003

90. Verma S, Szmitko PE, Ridker PM. C-reactive protein comes of age. Nat Clin Pract Cardiovasc 2005; 2: 29–36

91. Sakkinen P, Abbott RD, Curb JD, et al. C-reactive protein and myocardial infarction. J Clin Epidemiol 2002; 55: 445–51

92. Albert CM, Ma J, Rifai N, et al. Prospective study of C-reactive protein, homocysteine, and plasma lipid levels as predictors of sudden cardiac death. Circulation 2002; 105: 2595–9

93. Ridker PM, Rifai N, Pfeffer MA, et al. Inflammation, pravastatin, and the risk of coronary events after myocardial infarction in patients with average cholesterol levels. Cholesterol and Recurrent Events (CARE) Investigators. Circulation 1998; 98: 839–44

94. Ridker PM, Cushman M, Stampfer MJ, et al. Inflammation, aspirin, and the risk of cardiovascular disease in apparently healthy men. N Engl J Med 1997; 336: 973–9

95. Pradhan AD, Manson JE, Rossouw JE, et al. Inflammatory biomarkers, hormone replacement therapy, and incident coronary heart disease: prospective analysis from the Women's Health Initiative observational study. JAMA 2002; 288: 980–7

96. Ridker PM. Role of inflammatory biomarkers in prediction of coronary heart disease. Lancet 2001; 358: 946–8

97. Ridker PM, Rifai N, Rose L, et al. Comparison of C-reactive protein and low-density lipoprotein cholesterol levels in the prediction of first cardiovascular events. N Engl J Med 2002; 347: 1557–65

98. Pradhan AD, Manson JE, Rifai N, et al. C-reactive protein, interleukin 6, and risk of developing type 2 diabetes mellitus. JAMA 2001; 286: 327–34

8 Managing cardiometabolic risk – a brief review

INTRODUCTION

As the rates of various cardiometabolic risk factors rise, new treatments for such diseases and conditions continue to proliferate. While the development of therapeutic agents to combat risk factors, such as obesity and diabetes, still lags behind the epidemic, there are a variety of current therapies, both pharmacological and other, to arm the clinician in the battle to reduce cardiometabolic risk. While a full review of all the available treatments for cardiometabolic risk is beyond the scope of this chapter and, indeed, this volume, what follows is a brief summary of major treatment modalities.

Diet and nutrition

It has long been recommended that a healthy diet is the foundation of therapy to modify cardiometabolic risk. The landmark trial of diet-based modification of blood pressure tested what has become known as the DASH (Dietary Approaches to Stop Hypertension) diet (fruits, vegetables, low-fat dairy products) in conjunction with lowering sodium intake to alter significantly both systolic and diastolic blood pressures[1]. Not only was there a significant 6.7 mmHg drop in systolic between the high and low sodium control diets, but adding the DASH diet boosted that effect (Figure 8.1).

Diets balanced with protein or unsaturated fats, such as those in the Optimal Macronutrient Intake Trial for Heart Health (OMNIHEART)[2], also demonstrated the ability to modify factors such as blood pressure and low-density lipoprotein (LDL). One hundred and sixty-four participants in either intervention arm (protein modified or unsaturated fat modified), versus those in the standard carbohydrate diet group, exhibited a greater decrease in systolic blood pressure and LDL despite there being no difference in weight loss among the three groups. Figure 8.2 shows the food guide pyramid for a balanced diet[3]. In 2005, Dansinger et al. compared four 'fad' diets, the Atkins, Ornish, Weight Watchers, and Zone diets, in a randomized trial of 160 participants[4]. They found that each had a similar, mild effect on weight, as well as other cardiometabolic risk factors such as LDL/high-density lipoprotein (HDL) ratio and C-reactive protein (CRP) (tied to the weight loss effects). This attenuated effect was probably the result of poor long-term compliance with the diets across the board (Table 8.1).

In a recent publication, the Women's Health Initiative randomized nearly 50 000 women to intense dietary counseling to reduce dietary fat intake and increase fruits and vegetables versus the comparison group that received educational materials[5]. The trial did not demonstrate a significant effect on cardiovascular end points over a mean of 8 years of follow-up, in part because of only modest improvement in diet in the intervention group. Thus, compliance remains the key barrier (Figure 8.3).

Exercise and weight loss

Like diet, exercise and weight loss have also been associated with lower cardiometabolic risk factors; however, these interventions are equally difficult to sustain

Table 8.1 Changes in weight and cardiac risk factors in an analysis in which baseline values were carried forward in the case of missing data[*]. From reference 4, with permission

Variable	Diet group, mean change (SD)				p Value for trend across diets
	Atkins (n = 40)	Zone (n = 40)	Weight watchers (n = 40)	Ornish (n = 40)	
Weight (kg)					
2 mo	−3.6 (3.3)[†]	−3.8 (3.6)[†]	−3.5 (3.8)[†]	−3.6 (3.4)[†]	0.89
6 mo	−3.2 (4.9)[†]	−3.4 (5.7)[†]	−3.5 (5.6)[†]	−3.6 (6.7)[†]	0.76
12 mo	−2.1 (4.8)[†]	−3.2 (6.0)[†]	−3.0 (4.9)[‡]	−3.3 (7.3)[†]	0.40
BMI					
2 mo	−1.3 (1.1)[†]	−1.3 (1.2)[†]	−1.2 (1.3)[†]	−1.2 (1.1)[†]	0.83
6 mo	−1.1 (1.7)[†]	−0.9 (2.4)[‡]	−1.2 (2.0)[†]	−1.2 (2.3)[†]	0.65
12 mo	−0.7 (1.6)[†]	−1.1 (2.0)[†]	−1.1 (1.7)[†]	−1.4 (2.5)[‡]	0.36
Waist circumference (cm)					
2 mo	−3.3 (3.1)[†]	−3.0 (3.5)[†]	−3.5 (4.2)[†]	−2.7 (3.2)[†]	0.37
6 mo	−3.2 (4.9)[†]	−2.9 (5.2)[†]	−3.5 (5.9)[†]	−2.5 (5.3)[†]	0.69
12 mo	−2.5 (4.5)[†]	−2.9 (5.3)[†]	−3.3 (5.4)[†]	−2.2 (5.5)[‡]	0.89
Total cholesterol (mg/dL)					
2 mo	−1.8 (24)	−18.4 (25)[†]	−14.8 (26)[†]	−19.0 (28)[†]	0.01
6 mo	−0.9 (18)	−6.2 (19)[‡]	−8.1 (21)[‡]	−11.4 (26)[†]	0.03
12 mo	−4.3 (23)	−10.1 (35)	−8.2 (24)[‡]	−10.8 (21)[†]	0.35
LDL cholesterol (mg/dL)					
2 mo	1.3 (18)	−9.7 (27)[‡]	−12.1 (25)[†]	−16.5 (25)[†]	0.001
6 mo	−2.7 (14)	−6.7 (22)	−7.0 (24)	−10.5 (22)[†]	0.10
12 mo	−7.1 (24)	−11.8 (34)[‡]	−9.3 (27)[‡]	−12.6 (19)[†]	0.46
HDL cholesterol (mg/dL)					
2 mo	3.2 (6.2)[†]	1.8 (7.6)	−0.2 (11.8)	−3.6 (7.3)[†]	0.001
6 mo	3.8 (6.4)[†]	3.6 (10.5)[‡]	2.4 (9.0)	−1.5 (7.0)	0.005
12 mo	3.4 (7.1)[†]	3.3 (10.3)[‡]	3.4 (9.9)[‡]	−0.5 (6.5)	0.06
Total/HDL cholesterol ratio					
2 mo	−0.36 (0.66)[†]	−0.66 (1.06)[†]	−0.49 (1.86)	−0.18 (1.01)	0.40
6 mo	−0.38 (0.68)[†]	−0.46 (0.93)[†]	−0.60 (1.57)[‡]	−0.25 (1.07)	0.75
12 mo	−0.39 (0.69)[†]	−0.52 (1.04)[†]	−0.70 (1.67)[‡]	−0.30 (0.96)	0.89
LDL/HDL cholesterol ratio					
2 mo	−0.18 (0.57)	−0.33 (0.79)[†]	−0.42 (1.55)	−0.21 (0.67)	0.81
6 mo	−0.30 (0.55)[†]	−0.30 (0.74)[†]	−0.47 (1.37)[‡]	−0.22 (0.70)	0.90
12 mo	−0.39 (0.81)[†]	−0.40 (0.81)[†]	−0.55 (1.39)[‡]	−0.31 (0.68)[†]	0.92
Triglycerides (mg/dL)					
2 mo	−32.3 (66)[†]	−54.1 (105)[†]	−9.2 (39)	−0.4 (77)	0.01
6 mo	−10.6 (40)	−14.8 (57)	−1.5 (55)	−2.3 (71)	0.35
12 mo	−1.2 (84)	2.5 (147)	−12.7 (61)	5.6 (36)	0.93
Systolic BP (mmHg)					
2 mo	−4.2 (13)[‡]	−4.1 (14)	−4.8 (13)[‡]	−1.3 (8.8)	0.19
6 mo	−3.7 (10)[‡]	−3.9 (14)	−4.8 (14)[‡]	−0.6 (8.7)	0.32
12 mo	−0.2 (12)	1.4 (15)	−2.7 (13)	0.5 (7.7)	0.71
Diastolic BP (mmHg)					
2 mo	−4.2 (8.3)[†]	−4.8 (7.6)[†]	−3.1 (7.4)[‡]	−2.5 (7.1)[‡]	0.19
6 mo	−4.0 (6.5)[†]	−4.0 (9.1)[†]	−1.8 (6.9)	−0.3 (6.2)	0.01
12 mo	−1.4 (7.5)	−1.2 (9.5)	−1.7 (6.4)	0.2 (4.6)	0.40
Glucose (mg/dL)					
2 mo	−9.8 (30)[‡]	−9.0 (29)	−5.5 (24)	−3.1 (23)	0.21
6 mo	−7.8 (26)	−8.2 (33)	−3.8 (22)	−5.1 (25)	0.50
12 mo	1.4 (30)	−4.2 (18)	−4.7 (19)	−4.1 (30)	0.34
Insulin (μIU/mL)					
2 mo	−5.1 (13)[†]	−7.1 (12)[†]	−1.8 (6.0)	−1.7 (12)	0.06
2 mo	−2.3 (11)	−1.9 (16)	−2.5 (7.1)	−0.4 (18)	0.60
12 mo	−1.2 (6.7)	−5.4 (14)[†]	−2.6 (6.1)[†]	−3.0 (6.3)[‡]	0.70
C-reactive protein (mg/L)					
2 mo	−0.33 (1.6)	−0.22 (1.9)	−0.04 (1.2)	−0.61 (2.6)	0.61
6 mo	−0.71 (2.0)[‡]	−0.42 (1.9)	−0.50 (1.5)[‡]	−0.70 (2.8)	0.97
12 mo	−0.70 (2.1)[‡]	−0.58 (2.1)	−0.58 (1.3)[†]	−0.88 (2.4)[‡]	0.70

BMI, body mass index (calculated as weight in kilograms divided by the square of height in meters); BP, blood pressure; HDL, high-density lipoprotein; LDL, low-density lipoproteins; mo, months. SI conversions: to convert glucose to mmol/L, multiply by 0.0555; HDL, LDL, and total cholesterol to mmol/L, multiply by 0.0259; insulin to pmol/L, multiply by 6.945; and triglycerides to mmol/L, multiply by 0.0113. *For Atkins group, the actual numbers of records available were 31 at 2 months, 22 at 6 months, and 21 at 12 months; for Zone group, 33 at 2 months, 26 at 6 months, and 26 at 12 months; for Weight Watchers group, 33 at 2 months, 30 at 6 months, and 26 at 12 months; for Ornish group, 29 at 2 months, 21 at 6 months, and 20 at 12 months.

[†]p < 0.01 for difference from baseline within the group.
[‡]p < 0.05 for difference from baseline within the group

Table 8.2 Barriers to weight loss and increased physical activity. From reference 6, with permission

Barrier	Possible solution
Personal	
Lack of perceived benefits	Explain hazards of overweight and sedentary lifestyle including potential years of life lost as well as benefits of weight control and physical activity
Lack of time	Advise patient that accumulation of short periods of activity each day is an alternative to lengthy periods; healthy eating need not take more time than unhealthy eating
Lack of motivation	Write a 'prescription' for weight loss or increased physical activity, help patient set realistic initial goals, and monitor progress
Lack of support	Encourage patient to schedule physical activity with a partner, friend, or club at work; schedule follow-up visits to monitor progress
Environmental	
Lack of access to exercise facilities, concerns about neighborhood safety	Compile and distribute a list of local centers that offer exercise facilities: community centers, YMCA/YWCAs, educational institutions, etc.
Built environment	Take part in the CDC and Prevention's Active Community Environments program
Lack of healthy food or physical education in schools	As a physician-citizen, encourage the school board to offer healthier choices in school lunches and maintain or increase daily activity time

over long periods of time. In a 'call to action,' Manson *et al.* demonstrated both the advantages and barriers to weight loss, and provided a good approach to conquering those barriers and realizing the benefits. They recommend diet, physical activity, and behavioral therapy to achieve weight loss in those with a body mass index (BMI) between 25 and 27, and pharmacotherapy for patients with a BMI up to 30 or with co-morbidities[6]. Bariatric surgery is only recommended for patients with a BMI over 40, or > 35 for those with co-morbidities (Tables 8.2–8.4)[6].

Pharmacotherapy to reduce body weight has also demonstrated a concurrent improvement in biochemical marking of cardiometabolic risk. Sibutramine, a weight loss agent that speeds satiety and increases basal metabolic rate by inhibiting uptake of the neurotransmitters noradrenaline and serotonin, was tested in a randomized placebo-controlled trial of 1002 obese patients over 44 weeks. Over this period, an improvement in lipid profile concurrent with sibutramine's weight loss effects was demonstrated (Figure 8.4)[7].

Trials of the new endocannabinoid antagonist, rimonabant, have also provided good evidence of its ability to modify cardiometabolic risk factors through both weight loss and effects independent of weight change. In several trials of over 1000 overweight patients, the Rimonabant In Obesity (RIO) program

Table 8.3 Possible elements for a 'prescription' for increased physical activity. From reference 6, with permission

Physical activity

Take the stairs whenever possible

Purchase a pedometer, aim for 10 000 steps per day

Display 'exercise prescription' in a visible place

If you drive to work or stores, park in a space far away from the door and walk

If you take public transportation, get off a stop early and walk

Walk on your lunch break

Try exercising with friends or a group

Consider strength training for 20 min 2–3 times per week

Table 8.4 Possible elements for a 'prescription' for weight loss or maintenance. From reference 6, with permission

Nutrition

Pay attention to portions; avoid supersizing; when eating out, consider splitting an entrée

Set regular times to eat: 3 meals and no more than 2 snacks per day

Limit saturated and *trans* fats

Increase daily intake of fruit and vegetables: at least 5, aim for 7–9

Since fiber can increase the feeling of fullness, aim for 2–3 servings of whole grain food per day

Limit sweetened beverages, drink water, or non-fat or 1% milk

Table 8.5 Rates of continuous smoking abstinence in two studies comparing varenicline, bupropion, and placebo. Weeks 9–12, primary end point; weeks 9–52, secondary end point. From reference 12, with permission

Parameter	Varenicline	Bupropion	Placebo
Study 1	n = 349	n = 329	n = 344
Rate (%), OR, p value*			
weeks 9–12	44.4	29.5, 1.96, < 0.0001	17.7, 3.91, < 0.0001
weeks 9–52	22.1	16.4, 1.45, 0.064	8.4, 3.13, < 0.0001
Study 2	n = 343	n = 340	n = 340
Rate (%), OR, p value*			
weeks 9–12	44.0	30.0, 1.89, < 0.0001	17.7, 3.85, < 0.0001
weeks 9–52	23.0	15.0, 1.72, < 0.0001	10.3, 2.66, < 0.0001

*OR and p value compared with varenicline

demonstrated dose–response improvements not only in weight loss, but also in other risk factors such as LDL, HDL, and triglycerides. These effects were commonly significant at 1 year of follow-up[8–10].

There is one caveat to the trials involving pharmacological agents for weight loss: they predominantly include patients who are obese or morbidly obese. Thus, the effects of these medications and their abilities to improve cardiometabolic risk in persons of normal to slightly overweight body habitus are largely unknown.

Smoking cessation

While many patients are aware of its dangers and can quit smoking for a period, it takes an average of three attempts to quit successfully in the long term. However, this is well worth it, as the reduction in mortality is substantial, and has been consistently demonstrated across studies. In 2003, Critchley and Capewell reviewed outcomes of over 12 000 patients in trials of smoking cessation to quantify a 36% relative risk reduction of mortality for those patients who quit smoking (Figure 8.5)[11].

New agents are also in the pipeline to assist in this challenge, including varenicline, a new nicotine receptor blocker. It proved superior to bupropion in terms of abstainers at the 3- and 12-month marks (Table 8.5)[12]. However, the absolute percentages of patients who had abstained for a full 12 months (23% in the varenicline group vs. 15% for bupropion) was still low overall, demonstrating both the difficulty of successfully intervening and the progress that has yet to be made in smoking cessation therapies.

Antiplatelet therapy

Antiplatelet therapies, the cornerstone of pharmacological cardiovascular prevention, play a vital role in minimizing events, although they do not actually modify an individual's cardiovascular risk factors.

Aspirin has long been found significantly to reduce a host of events, with the expected effect magnification in more high-risk patients. This was quantified in a meta-analysis by Hayden *et al.*, which identified a 28% reduction in non-fatal MI or coronary death, and statistically non-significant trends towards reducing coronary disease mortality, stroke, and all-cause mortality in the primary prevention setting (Figure 8.6)[13]. Following the large placebo-controlled trials for primary prevention, the Antithrombotic Trialists' Collaboration reviewed 195 trials of more than 135 000 patients. They identified not only benefits in both primary and secondary prevention across subgroups, but also found little benefit associated with daily aspirin at doses below 75 mg. (Figure 8.7)[14].

The role of aspirin in secondary prevention of cardiovascular events was demonstrated in the PARIS II[15]. The daily dose of aspirin was further refined based on the bleeding incidence results of the Clopidogrel in Unstable angina to prevent Recurrent Events (CURE) trial[16]. They found a dose-response of major bleeding with aspirin at daily doses above 100 mg (Figure 8.8)[16].

An alternative platelet agent, clopidogrel, is an irreversible inhibitor of the P2Y12 ADP receptor on platelets. Several trials have demonstrated its role as either a replacement for, or an adjunctive to, aspirin in various clinical settings. The Clopidogrel versus

Table 8.6 Results of the CHARISMA trial: primary and secondary end points comparing clopidogrel aspirin versus aspirin alone. From reference 21, with permission

End point	Clopidogrel plus Aspirin $n = 7802$ (n (%))	Placebo plus Aspirin $n = 7801$ (n (%))	Relative risk (95% CI)	p Value
Efficacy end points				
Primary efficacy end points	534 (6.8)	573 (7.3)	0.93 (0.83–1.05)	0.22
Death from any cause	371 (4.8)	374 (4.8)	0.99 (0.86–1.14)	0.90
Death from cardiovascular cause	238 (3.1)	229 (2.9)	1.04 (0.87–1.25)	0.68
Myocardial infarction (non-fatal)	147 (1.9)	159 (2.0)	0.92 (0.74–1.16)	0.48
Ischemic stroke (non-fatal)	132 (1.7)	160 (2.1)	0.82 (0.66–1.04)	0.10
Stroke (non-fatal)	149 (1.9)	185 (2.4)	0.80 (0.65–0.997)	0.05
Secondary efficacy end point	1301 (16.7)	1395 (17.9)	0.92 (0.86–0.995)	0.04
Hospitalization for unstable angina, transient ischemic attack, or revascularization	866 (11.1)	957 (12.3)	0.90 (0.82–0.98)	0.02
Safety end points				
Severe bleeding	130 (1.7)	104 (1.3)	1.25 (0.97–1.61)	0.09
Fatal bleeding	26 (0.3)	17 (0.2)	1.53 (0.83–2.82)	0.17
Primary intracranial hemorrhage	26 (0.3)	27 (0.3)	0.96 (0.56–1.65)	0.89
Moderate bleeding	164 (2.1)	101 (1.3)	1.62 (1.62–2.10)	< 0.001

CI, confidence inteval
The secondary efficacy end point was the first occurrence of myocardial infarction, stroke, death from cardiovascular cause, or hospitilization for unstable angina, a transient ischemic attack, or a revascularization procedure (coronary, cerebral, or peripheral)

Aspirin in Patients at Risk of Ischaemic Events (CAPRIE) trial randomized over 19 000 patients with some manifestation of atherosclerotic disease to receive either aspirin or clopidogrel, with a mean follow-up of almost 2 years. By reducing the risk of MI, ischemic stroke, or vascular death, the trial established clopidogrel's superiority to aspirin in preventing recurrent ischemic events in this high-risk population (Figure 8.9)[17].

The CURE[18], CLARITY-TIMI 28[19], and COMMIT[20] trials collectively randomized approximately 62 000 patients with acute coronary syndromes to receive either clopidogrel or placebo in addition to usual therapies (Figures 8.10–8.12). They demonstrated the superiority of treatment with clopidogrel for both clinical and angiographic end points in durations of up to 1 year, and that these benefits were maximized with earlier treatment. However the Clopidogrel for High Atherothrombic Risk and Ischemic Stabilization, Management and Avoidance (CHARISMA)

trial failed to demonstrate the use of clopidogrel in the primary prevention setting (Table 8.6)[21].

Statin therapy

As the role of LDL cholesterol in atherothrombotic events became clear and, subsequently, 3-hydroxy-3-methylglutaryl coenzyme A (HMG-CoA) reductase inhibitors (statins) to lower LDL were developed, several trials demonstrated the impressive translation of pharmacotherapy lowering LDL to a reduction in atherosclerosis and clinical event rates (Figure 8.13). Placebo-controlled trials, for both primary and secondary prevention, have been summarized in the Cholesterol Treatment Trialists' (CTT) meta-analysis (Figures 8.14–8.16)[23]. This collective experience of 90 000 patients in 14 randomized trials demonstrated a significant 12% reduction in all-cause mortality for every mmol/L (~38 mg/dL) reduction of LDL, significant within the first year of treatment. The highly significant reductions in vascular events were roughly

20–30% and maintained significance across subgroups. This was true even for patients who started in the lowest range of LDL levels (≤ 3.5 mmol/L or ~133 mg/dL), as well as those with higher LDL values. These findings were consistent with the 2002 Heart Protection Study, which not only confirmed the benefit of statins in secondary prevention, but also demonstrated a treatment effect even for those patients with an LDL below 3.0 mmol/L (116 mg/dL) at the time of randomization (Figure 8.17)[24]. The Collaborative Atorvastatin Diabetes Study (CARDS) also verified the primary preventive value of statins in patients with low LDL (~120 mg/dL); they randomized nearly 4000 high-risk type 2 diabetic patients to either placebo or low-dose atorvastatin. The primary end point of acute coronary syndrome, coronary revascularization, or stroke was met at a median follow-up of 3.9 years, 2 years earlier than the design of the trial had anticipated (Figure 8.18)[25].

This begged the critical question: how low should we go? Subsequently, trials of high- versus standard-dose statins, such as PROVE IT-TIMI 22, yielded median LDL levels in the two treatment arms (atorvastatin 80 mg vs. pravastatin 40 mg) of 62 and 95 mg/dL, respectively. This difference proved that there was a significant benefit of continued lowering of LDL to reduce clinical cardiovascular events (Figure 8.19)[26]. However, the benefits of statins extend beyond lowering LDL, as they have also been shown, in several trials, to reduce C-reactive protein (CRP), a known inflammatory marker for atherosclerotic disease.

Fibrates

Raising HDL and triglyceride lowering with the use of fenofibrate has also been demonstrated to affect clinical events, although to a lesser extent than LDL lowering. The Veterans Affairs High-density lipoprotein cholesterol Intervention Trial (VAHIT) of 2531 patients found that gemfibrozil was associated with a 20% reduction in the risk of death or MI[27]. The Fenofibrate Intervention and Event Lowering in Diabetes (FIELD) trial randomized almost 10 000 diabetics who were not taking a statin to receive fenofibrate or placebo (Figure 8.20)[28]. After an average of 5 years of follow-up, reduction in the primary end point of coronary death or MI was not significant despite a signifi-

Table 8.7 Benefit of antihypertensive treatment Data from the VA Cooperative Study, 1967: assessable morbid/fatal events. From reference 36, with permission

	Placebo $n = 70$	Active treatment* $n = 73$
Accelerated hypertension	12	0
Stroke	4	1
Coronary event	2	0
Congestive heart failure	2	0
Renal damage	2	0
Deaths	4	0

*$p < 0.001$ active antihypertensive therapy vs. placebo

cant 24% reduction in non-fatal MI alone. However, the treatment effect of fenofibrate raised HDL only marginally compared with placebo, and significantly more patients in the placebo arm than in the fenofibrate arm began statin therapy during the trial. Thus, it is possible that interventions with greater treatment effects on HDL could yield more convincing clinical results.

Diabetes

Historically, strict blood glucose control in diabetics was only shown to reduce or delay the onset of microvascular disease such as retinopathy and neuropathy (Figures 8.21, 8.22 and 8.23)[29]. The UK Prospective Diabetes Study (UKPDS) compared conventional glucose control (fasting glucose < 15 mmol/L) with an intensive strategy (< 6 mmol/L) in over 4000 patients. Early data demonstrated the relationship between glycosylated hemoglobin (HbA1c) and microvascular events, and also hinted at a relationship with acute myocardial infarction rates (Figures 8.24–8.26)[30]. However, more recently the Diabetes Control and Complications Trial/Epidemiology of Diabetes Interventions and Complications (DCCT/EDIC) Study compared conventional treatment (preventing symptoms of hypoglycemia or hyperglycemia) with intensive glucose control (glucose 3.9–6.7 mmol/L and HbA1c < 6.05%)[32]. They demonstrated that, in 1400 patients over 17 years of follow-up (but a mean treatment period of 6.5 years), type 1 diabetics with stricter glucose control had lower rates of major cardiovascular events (cardiovascular death, any acute coronary syndrome, stroke, revascularization) than those with conventional treatment (Figure 8.27)[32].

The above trials used either sulfonylureas or insulin to alter the cardiometabolic risk associated with glucose intolerance. However, another class of medications for diabetes, the thiazolidinediones (TZDs), can have a pleiotropic effect on cardiometabolic risk. The PROspective pioglitAzone Clinical Trial In macroVascular Events (PROactive) randomized 5200 high-risk type 2 diabetes patients to receive either pioglitazone or placebo for a mean of 34 months[33]. Pioglitazone was found to reduce the main secondary end point of death, non-fatal MI, or stroke, despite a non-significant reduction in the broader primary end point (Figure 8.28). In addition, both pioglitazone and rosiglitazone have also been found to reduce inflammatory biomarkers associated with cardiovascular disease, particularly CRP[34,35].

Hypertension

One of the earliest studies to demonstrate a clinical benefit of reducing blood pressure was the VA Cooperative Study, where patients in the treated arm had far fewer coronary, cerebral, or renal vascular events even in the small study size of 143 (Table 8.7)[36]. The next question raised was whether it mattered *how* the blood pressure was lowered: were newer calcium channel blockers and angiotensin converting enzyme (ACE) inhibitors better than older alpha-blockers and diuretics? In a quest to provide the answer, the Antihypertensive and Lipid-Lowering Treatment to Prevent Heart Attack Trial (ALLHAT) compared these four drugs in over 42 000 patients. After the doxazosin arm was terminated early due to its clear inferiority, the remaining three drugs proved equivalent in their abilities to reduce coronary death or non-fatal MI (Figure 8.29)[37]. Thus, the thiazide diuretics became the primary antihypertensive medication in uncomplicated patients. However, therapies for hypertension have continued to evolve, requiring re-evaluation of the newest agents. The Anglo-Scandinavian Cardiac Outcomes Trial-Blood Pressure Lowering Arm (ASCOT-BPLA) compared the combination of calcium channel blocker and ACE inhibitor (amlodipine ± perindopril) with a beta-blocker and diuretic (atenolol

± bendroflumethiazide) in over 19 000 patients (Figure 8.30)[37]. Unfortunately, the 10% reduction in the primary end point (coronary death or non-fatal MI) in the amlodipine/perindopril arm did not reach statistical significance when the trial was stopped early owing to a higher incidence of all-cause mortality in the beta-blocker and diuretic arm.

With regard to the question of how low the blood pressure should be, the Hypertension Optimal Treatment (HOT) trial enrolled almost 19 000 patients to determine the relationship between diastolic pressure reduction and clinical events. While the lowest rate of major cardiovascular events was at a mean diastolic pressure of 82.6 mmHg, there was no significant difference in events between the overall groups with diastolic pressures less than 90, 85, or 80 mmHg (Figure 8.31)[38]. However, those in the more sensitive diabetic subgroup exhibited a strong dose–response relationship suggesting a real, yet small, treatment effect (Figure 8.32)[39].

Eplerenone

A newer aldosterone-blocking antihypertensive, eplerenone, is more selective for the mineralocorticoid receptor than its older sibling spironolactone. The Eplerenone Post-Acute Myocardial Infarction Heart Failure Efficacy and SUrvival Study (EPHESUS) compared eplerenone with placebo in 6500 patients with acute MI complicated by left ventricular dysfunction. They demonstrated a reduction in cardiovascular death, MI, stroke, ventricular arrhythmia, or hospitalization for heart failure over a mean follow-up of 16 months (Figure 8.33)[40].

CONCLUSION

Just as the problem of increasing cardiometabolic risk is multifactorial, so must be the approach to treating it. The evidence briefly reviewed here demonstrates the effective pharmacological agents available to reduce biochemical markers and the risk of events. However, these therapies must be considered within the greater problem of rising obesity and its associated pathologies. Physicians must continue to emphasize that there remains no substitute for lifestyle modification to combat cardiometabolic risk.

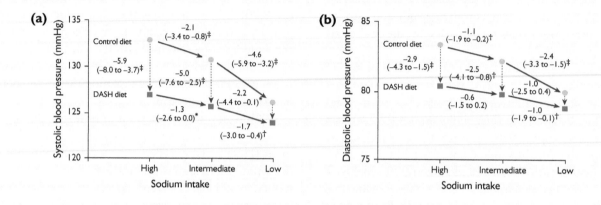

Figure 8.1 The effect on systolic blood pressure (a) and diastolic blood pressure (b) of reduced sodium intake and the DASH diet. *$p<0.05$; †$p<0.01$; ‡$p<0.001$. From reference 1, with permission

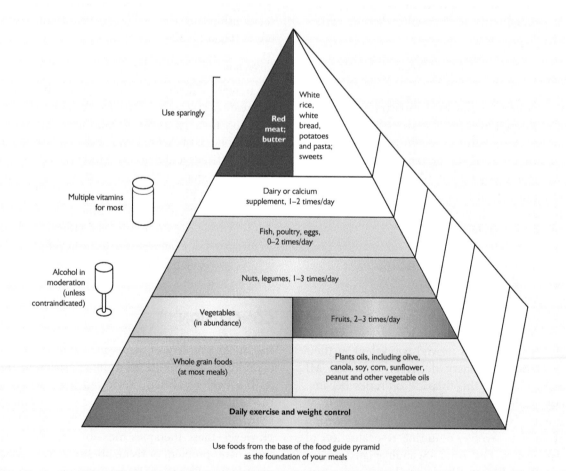

Figure 8.2 The food guide pyramid provides a structure for selecting foods. At the bottom are the whole grains, breads, and cereals. Above them are the fruits and vegetables, and above that the meats, cheese, and dairy products, with the recommended range of servings for each. From reference 3, with permission

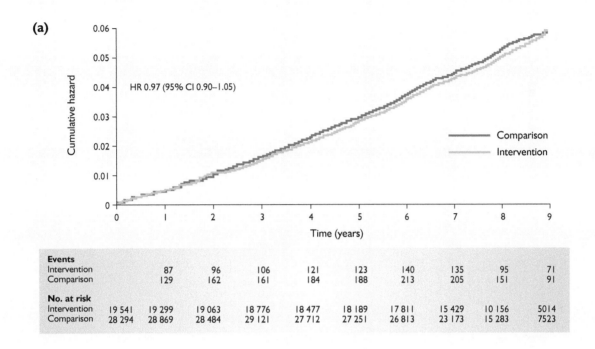

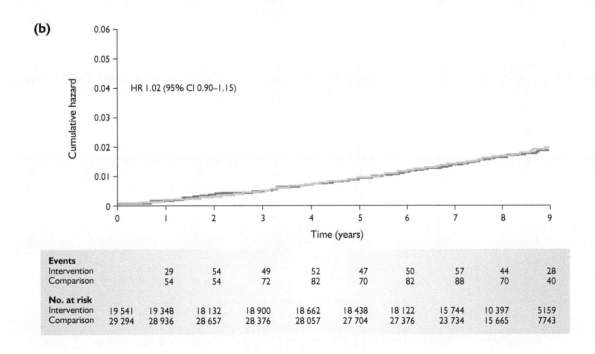

Figure 8.3 Effects of dietary intervention in the Women's Health Initiative. Kaplan–Meier estimates in all participants for myocardial infarction (MI), coronary heart disease (CHD), or revascularization (a) and for stroke (b), and in participants without a history of cardiovascular disease for MI, CHD, or revascularization (c) and for stroke (d). HR, hazard ratio; CI, confidence interval. From reference 5, with permission   *Continued*

(c)

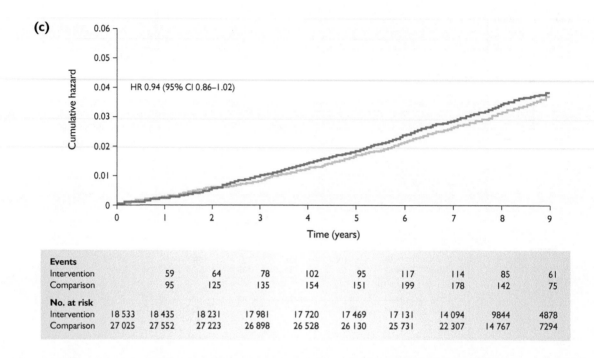

Events									
Intervention		59	64	78	102	95	117	114	85	61
Comparison		95	125	135	154	151	199	178	142	75
No. at risk									
Intervention	18 533	18 435	18 231	17 981	17 720	17 469	17 131	14 094	9844	4878
Comparison	27 025	27 552	27 223	26 898	26 528	26 130	25 731	22 307	14 767	7294

(d)

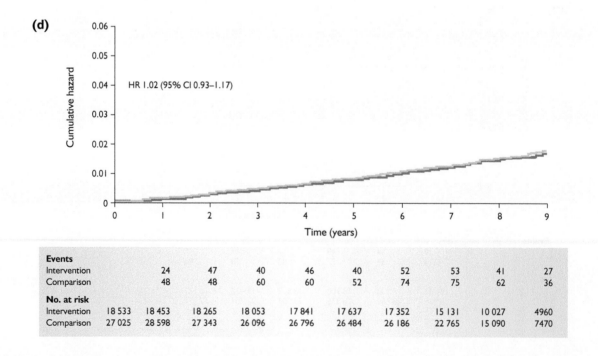

Events									
Intervention		24	47	40	46	40	52	53	41	27
Comparison		48	48	60	60	52	74	75	62	36
No. at risk									
Intervention	18 533	18 453	18 265	18 053	17 841	17 637	17 352	15 131	10 027	4960
Comparison	27 025	28 598	27 343	26 096	26 796	26 484	26 186	22 765	15 090	7470

Figure 8.3 *Continued*

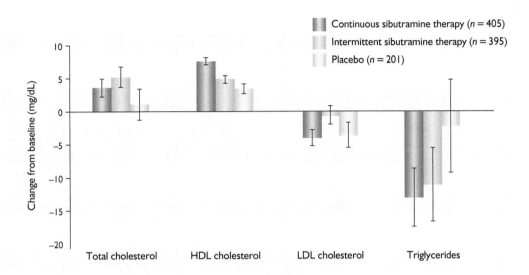

Figure 8.4 Difference in mean (SE) plasma lipid levels between placebo, continuous, and intermittent therapies with 15 mg of sibutramine hydrochloride. From reference 7, with permission

Study	Ceased smoking Patients (n)	Ceased smoking Deaths (n)	Continued smoking Patients (n)	Continued smoking Deaths (n)	Weight (%)	RR (95% CI)
Aberg et al., 1983	542	110	443	142	8.3	0.63 (0.51–0.79)
Baughman et al., 1982	45	9	32	14	1.8	0.46 (0.23–0.92)
Bednarzewski et al., 1984	455	136	555	205	9.3	0.81 (0.68–0.97)
Burr et al., 1992	665	27	521	41	3.5	0.52 (0.32–0.83)
Daly et al., 1983	217	80	157	129	9.0	0.45 (0.37–0.54)
Greenwood et al., 1995	396	64	138	29	4.5	0.76 (0.51–1.12)
Gupta et al., 1993	173	56	52	24	4.9	0.70 (0.49–1.01)
Halstrom et al., 1986	91	34	219	104	6.1	0.79 (0.58–1.06)
Hasdai et al., 1997	435	41	734	97	5.2	0.71 (0.50–1.01)
Hedback et al., 1993	83	31	74	40	5.2	0.69 (0.49–0.98)
Herlitz et al., 1995	115	20	102	31	3.2	0.57 (0.35–0.94)
Johansson et al., 1985	81	14	75	27	2.6	0.48 (0.27–0.84)
Perkins and Dick, 1985	52	9	67	30	2.1	0.39 (0.20–0.74)
Salonen, 1980	221	26	302	60	4.0	0.59 (0.39–0.91)
Sato et al., 1992	59	5	28	7	0.9	0.34 (0.12–0.97)
Sparrow and Dawber, 1978	56	10	139	40	2.3	0.62 (0.33–1.15)
Tofler et al., 1993	173	14	220	37	2.5	0.48 (0.27–0.86)
Van Domburg et al., 2000	238	109	318	202	9.8	0.72 (0.61–0.85)
Vietstra et al., 1986	1490	223	2675	586	10.4	0.68 (0.59–0.78)
Voors et al., 1996	72	26	95	37	4.4	0.93 (0.62–1.38)
Overall	5659	1044	6944	1884	100.00	0.64 (0.58–0.71)

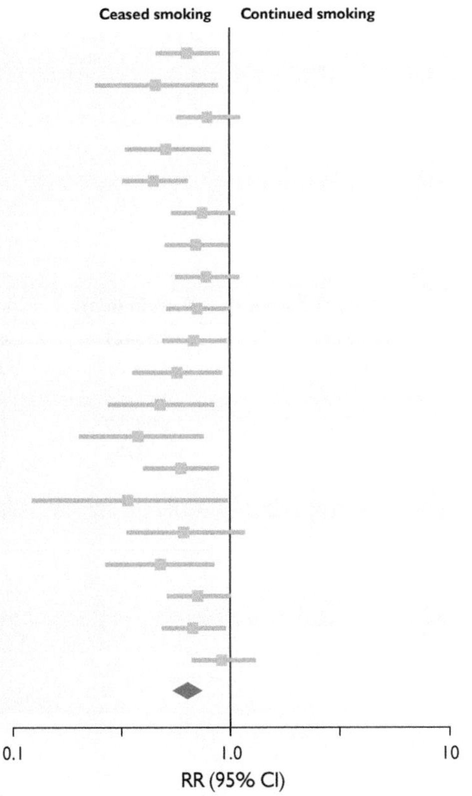

Ceased smoking   Continued smoking

0.1   1.0   10
RR (95% CI)

Figure 8.5 Pooled relative risks of mortality when patients with CHD stop smoking: random-effects meta-analysis of 20 studies. From reference 11, with permission

(a)

Study (reference)	Aspirin (n/n)	Control (n/n)	OR (95% CI random)	Weight (%)	OR (95% CI random)
BMD (5)	169/3429	88/1710		22.0	0.96 (0.73–1.24)
PHS (4)	163/11 037	266/11 034		27.8	0.61 (0.50–0.74)
TPT (7)	83/1268	107/1272		19.6	0.76 (0.57–1.03)
HOT (8)	82/9399	127/9391		20.9	0.64 (0.49–0.85)
PPP (9)	26/2226	35/2269		9.7	0.75 (0.45–1.26)
Total (95% CI)	523/27 359	623/25 676		100.0	0.72 (0.60–0.87)

0.20 0.50 1.0 2.0 5.0

Favors aspirin   Favors control

(b)

Study (reference)	Aspirin (n/n)	Control (n/n)	OR (95% CI random)	Weight (%)	OR (95% CI random)
BMD (5)	89/3429	47/1710		37.2	0.94 (0.66–1.35)
PHS (4)	34/11 037	53/11 034		25.6	0.64 (0.42–0.99)
TPT (7)	36/1268	34/1272		21.1	1.06 (0.66–1.71)
HOT (8)	14/9399	14/9391		8.7	1.00 (0.48–2.10)
PPP (9)	11/2226	13/2269		7.4	0.86 (0.39–1.93)
Total (95% CI)	184/27 359	161/25 676		100.0	0.87 (0.70–1.09)

0.20 0.50 1.0 2.0 5.0

Favors aspirin   Favors control

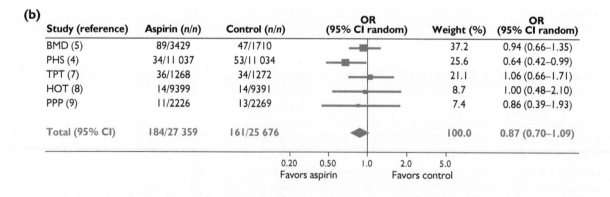

Figure 8.6 Meta-analysis of the effect of aspirin on total heart disease events (a), coronary heart disease mortality (b), fatal and non-fatal stroke events (c), and all-cause mortality (d). From reference 13, with permission   *Continued*

(c)

Study (reference)	Aspirin (n/n)	Control (n/n)	OR (95% CI random)	Weight (%)	OR (95% CI random)
BMD (5)	91/3429	39/1710		18.4	1.17 (0.80–1.71)
PHS (4)	119/11 037	98/11 034		29.8	1.22 (0.93–1.59)
TPT (7)	18/1268	26/1272		8.4	0.69 (0.38–1.27)
HOT (8)	146/9399	148/9391		35.6	0.99 (0.78–1.24)
PPP (9)	16/2226	24/2269		7.7	0.68 (0.36–1.28)
Total (95% CI)	390/27 359	335/25 676		100.0	1.02 (0.85–1.23)

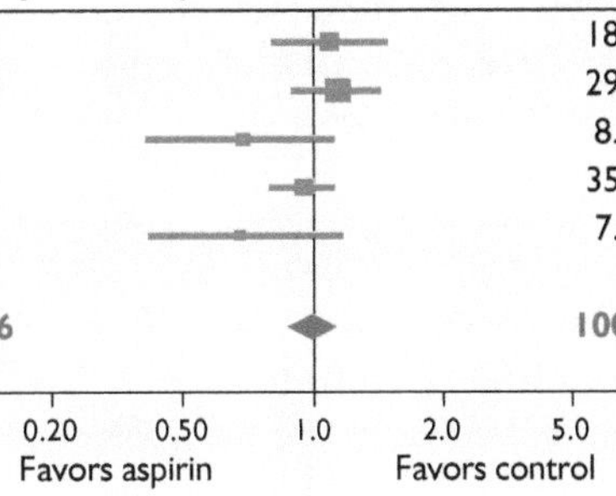

0.20   0.50   1.0   2.0   5.0
Favors aspirin   Favors control

(d)

Study (reference)	Aspirin (n/n)	Control (n/n)	OR (95% CI random)	Weight (%)	OR (95% CI random)
BMD (5)	270/3429	151/1710		20.9	0.88 (0.72–1.09)
PHS (4)	217/11 037	227/11 034		25.6	0.95 (0.79–1.15)
TPT (7)	113/1268	110/1272		12.0	1.03 (0.79–1.36)
HOT (8)	284/9399	305/9391		33.6	0.93 (0.79–1.09)
PPP (9)	62/2226	78/2269		7.9	0.80 (0.57–1.13)
Total (95% CI)	946/27 359	871/25 676		100.0	0.93 (0.84–1.02)

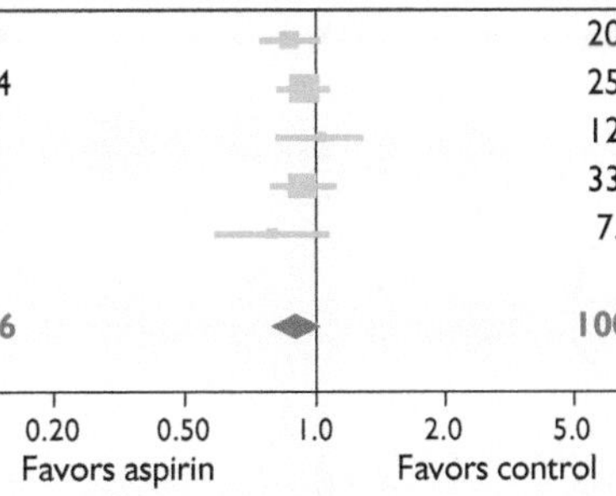

0.20   0.50   1.0   2.0   5.0
Favors aspirin   Favors control

Figure 8.6 *Continued*

Category of trial	No of trials with data	No (%) of vascular events		Observed–expected	Variance	Odds ratio (CI) Antiplatelet : control	% Odds reduction (SE)
		Allocated antiplatelet	Adjusted control				
Previous myocardial infarction	12	1345/9984 (13.5)	1708/10022 (17.0)	−159.8	567.6		25 (4)
Acute myocardial infarction	15	1007/9658 (10.4)	1370/9644 (14.2)	−181.5	519.2		30 (4)
Previous stroke/transient ischemic attack	21	2045/11493 (17.8)	2464/11527 (21.4)	−152.1	625.8		22 (4)
Acute stroke	7	1670/20418 (8.2)	1858/20403 (9.1)	−94.6	795.3		11 (3)
Other high risk	140	1638/20359 (8.0)	2102/20543 (10.2)	−222.3	737.0		26 (3)
Subtotal: all except acute stroke	188	6035/51494 (11.7)	7644/51736 (14.8)	−715.7	2449.6		25 (2)
All trials	195	7705/71912 (10.7)	9502/72139 (13.2)	−810.3	3244.9		22 (2)

Heterogeneity of odds reductions between:

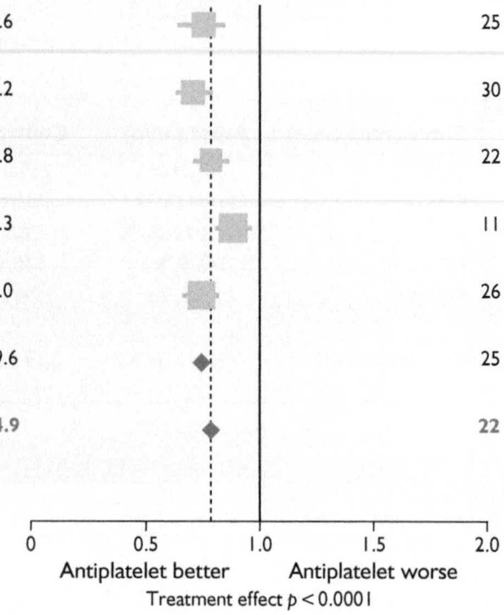

0   0.5   1.0   1.5   2.0
Antiplatelet better   Antiplatelet worse
Treatment effect p < 0.0001

Figure 8.7 Data from the Antithrombotic Trialists' Collaboration (ATC) demonstrating the efficacy of antiplatelet therapy on myocardial infarction, stroke, or vascular death. From reference 14, with permission

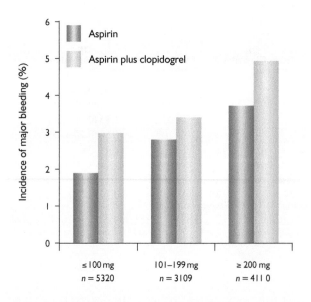

Figure 8.8 Aspirin dose and the incidence of major bleeding. From reference 16, with permission

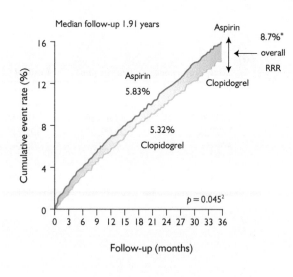

Figure 8.9 Efficacy of clopidogrel compared with aspirin in myocardial infarction, ischemic stroke, or vascular death in 19185 patients at risk of ischemic events. Annual rate of events is shown. *ITT (intention to treat) analysis. From reference 17, with permission

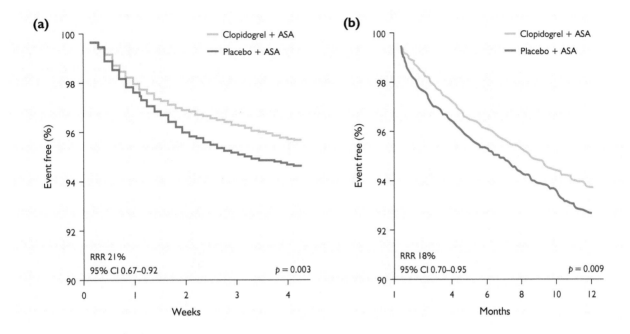

Figure 8.10 Data from the Clopidogrel in Unstable angina to prevent Recurrent Events trial demonstrating the benefit of clopidogrel therapy compared with placebo on cardiovascular death, stroke, or myocardial infarction within the first 1–30 days (a) and from 31 days to 1 year (b) of treatment in patients with unstable angina or non-ST elevation myocardial infarction. ASA, acetylsalicylic acid; RRR, relative risk ratio. From reference 18, with permission

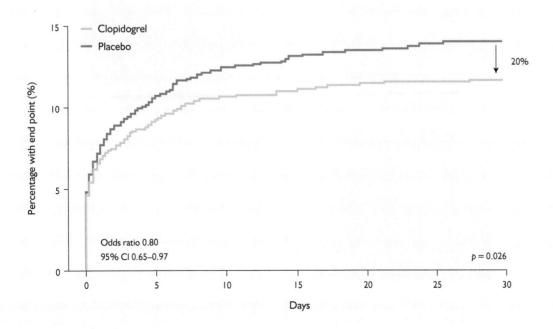

Figure 8.11 Efficacy of clopidogrel in reducing cardiovascular death, myocardial infarction or urgent revascularization compared with placebo in patients with ST elevation myocardial infarction treated with thrombolysis. From reference 19, with permission

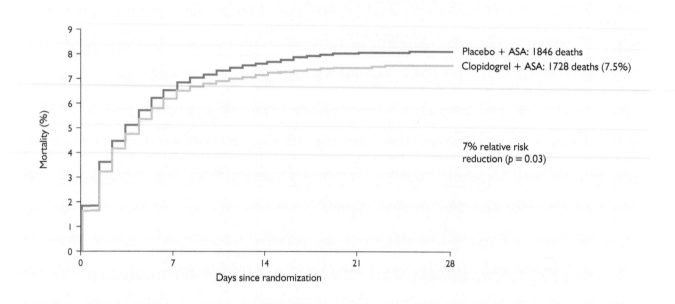

Figure 8.12 Effect of clopidogrel on death in patients with acute ST elevation myocardial infarction. ASA, acetylsalicylic acid. From reference 20, with permission

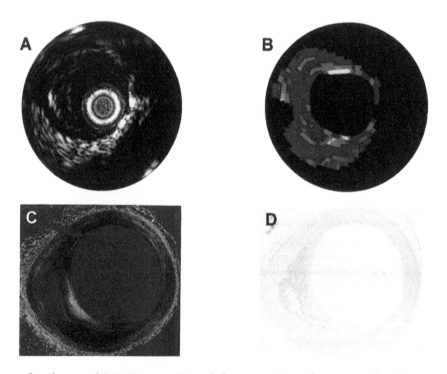

Figure 8.13 Intravascular ultrasound (IVUS) image (A) and elastogram (B) with corresponding histology of a coronary artery with a vulnerable plaque. The IVUS image reveals an eccentric plaque between the 6- and 12-o'clock positions. The elastogram shows high-strain regions (yellow) at the shoulders of the plaque surrounded by low-strain values (blue). The histology reveals a plaque with a typical vulnerable appearance: a thin cap with a lack of collagen at the shoulders (C) and a large atheroma with heavy infiltration of macrophages (D). From reference 22, with permission

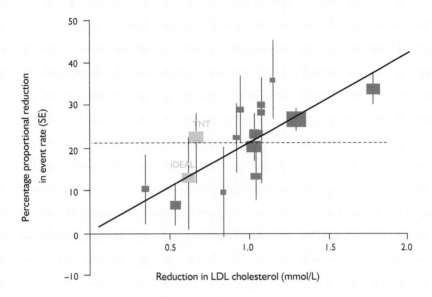

Figure 8.14 Cholesterol Treatment Trialists' collaboration showing the effects of statins on mortality per mmol/L LDL cholesterol reduction. Adapted from reference 23, with permission

End point	Events (%)		RR (CI) (Treatment : control)	Rate ratio (CI)
	Treatment	Control		
Non-fatal MI	2001 (4.4)	2769 (6.2)		0.74 (0.70–0.79)
CHD death	1548 (3.4)	1960 (4.4)		0.81 (0.75–0.87)
Any major coronary event	**3337 (7.4)**	**4420 (9.8)**		**0.77 (0.74–0.80)**
CABG	713 (3.3)	1006 (4.7)		0.75 (0.69–0.82)
PTCA	510 (2.4)	658 (3.1)		0.79 (0.69–0.90)
Unspecified	1397 (3.1)	1770 (3.9)		**0.76 (0.69–0.84)**
Any coronary revascularization	**2620 (5.8)**	**3434 (7.6)**		**0.76 (0.73–0.80)**
Hemorrhagic stroke	105 (0.2)	99 (0.2)		1.05 (0.78–1.41)
Presumed ischemic stroke	1235 (2.8)	1518 (3.4)		**0.81 (0.74–0.89)**
Any stroke	**1340 (3.0)**	**1617 (3.7)**		**0.83 (0.78–0.88)**
Any major vascular event	**6354 (14.1)**	**7994 (17.8)**		**0.79 (0.77–0.81)**
				$p < 0.0001$

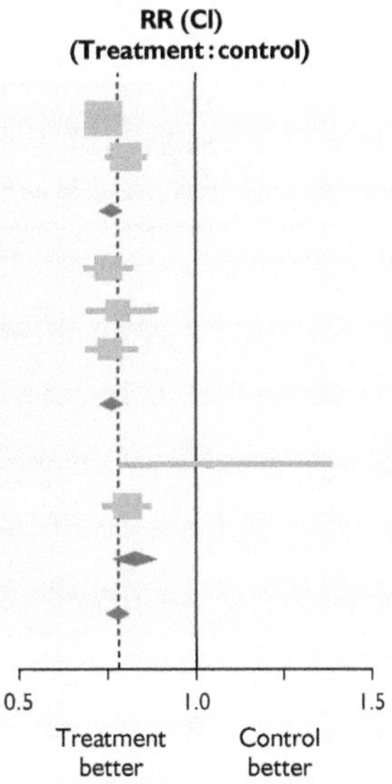

0.5   1.0   1.5

Treatment better   Control better

Figure 8.15 Cholesterol Treatment Trialists' collaboration showing the effects of statins on major vascular events. MI, myocardial infarction; CABG, coronary artery bypass graft; PTCA, percutaneous transluminal coronary angioplasty. Diamonds, summary; squares, data. From reference 23, with permission

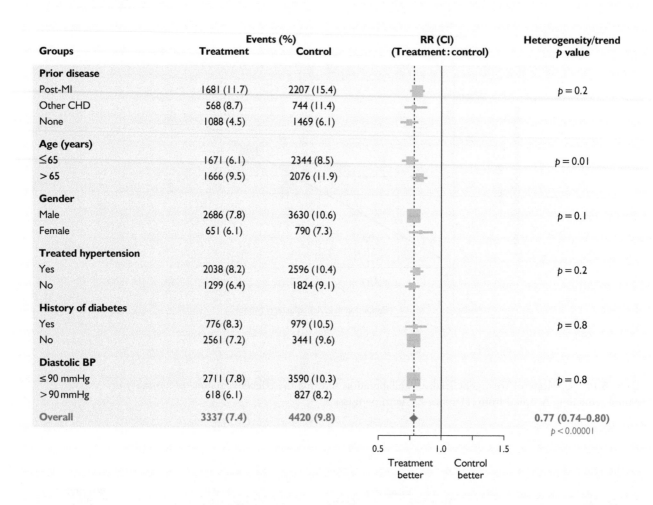

Groups	Events (%)		RR (CI) (Treatment : control)	Heterogeneity/trend p value
	Treatment	Control		
Prior disease				
Post-MI	1681 (11.7)	2207 (15.4)		p = 0.2
Other CHD	568 (8.7)	744 (11.4)		
None	1088 (4.5)	1469 (6.1)		
Age (years)				
≤65	1671 (6.1)	2344 (8.5)		p = 0.01
>65	1666 (9.5)	2076 (11.9)		
Gender				
Male	2686 (7.8)	3630 (10.6)		p = 0.1
Female	651 (6.1)	790 (7.3)		
Treated hypertension				
Yes	2038 (8.2)	2596 (10.4)		p = 0.2
No	1299 (6.4)	1824 (9.1)		
History of diabetes				
Yes	776 (8.3)	979 (10.5)		p = 0.8
No	2561 (7.2)	3441 (9.6)		
Diastolic BP				
≤90 mmHg	2711 (7.8)	3590 (10.3)		p = 0.8
>90 mmHg	618 (6.1)	827 (8.2)		
Overall	3337 (7.4)	4420 (9.8)		0.77 (0.74–0.80) p < 0.00001

0.5   1.0   1.5

Treatment better   Control better

Figure 8.16 Cholesterol Treatment Trialists' collaboration showing the effects of statins on major coronary events subdivided by baseline prognostic factors. From reference 23, with permission

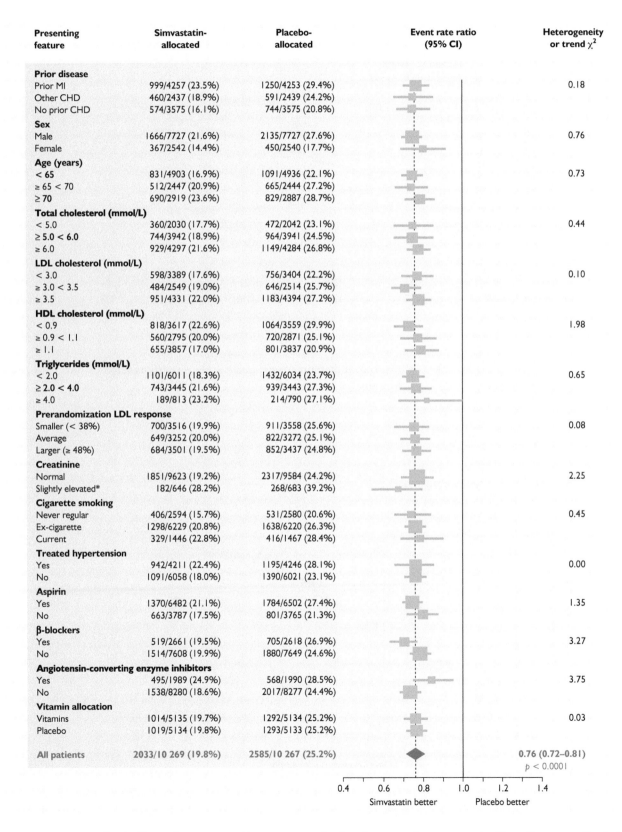

Presenting feature	Simvastatin-allocated	Placebo-allocated	Event rate ratio (95% CI)	Heterogeneity or trend χ^2
Prior disease				
Prior MI	999/4257 (23.5%)	1250/4253 (29.4%)		0.18
Other CHD	460/2437 (18.9%)	591/2439 (24.2%)		
No prior CHD	574/3575 (16.1%)	744/3575 (20.8%)		
Sex				
Male	1666/7727 (21.6%)	2135/7727 (27.6%)		0.76
Female	367/2542 (14.4%)	450/2540 (17.7%)		
Age (years)				
< 65	831/4903 (16.9%)	1091/4936 (22.1%)		0.73
≥ 65 < 70	512/2447 (20.9%)	665/2444 (27.2%)		
≥ 70	690/2919 (23.6%)	829/2887 (28.7%)		
Total cholesterol (mmol/L)				
< 5.0	360/2030 (17.7%)	472/2042 (23.1%)		0.44
≥ 5.0 < 6.0	744/3942 (18.9%)	964/3941 (24.5%)		
≥ 6.0	929/4297 (21.6%)	1149/4284 (26.8%)		
LDL cholesterol (mmol/L)				
< 3.0	598/3389 (17.6%)	756/3404 (22.2%)		0.10
≥ 3.0 < 3.5	484/2549 (19.0%)	646/2514 (25.7%)		
≥ 3.5	951/4331 (22.0%)	1183/4394 (27.2%)		
HDL cholesterol (mmol/L)				
< 0.9	818/3617 (22.6%)	1064/3559 (29.9%)		1.98
≥ 0.9 < 1.1	560/2795 (20.0%)	720/2871 (25.1%)		
≥ 1.1	655/3857 (17.0%)	801/3837 (20.9%)		
Triglycerides (mmol/L)				
< 2.0	1101/6011 (18.3%)	1432/6034 (23.7%)		0.65
≥ 2.0 < 4.0	743/3445 (21.6%)	939/3443 (27.3%)		
≥ 4.0	189/813 (23.2%)	214/790 (27.1%)		
Prerandomization LDL response				
Smaller (< 38%)	700/3516 (19.9%)	911/3558 (25.6%)		0.08
Average	649/3252 (20.0%)	822/3272 (25.1%)		
Larger (≥ 48%)	684/3501 (19.5%)	852/3437 (24.8%)		
Creatinine				
Normal	1851/9623 (19.2%)	2317/9584 (24.2%)		2.25
Slightly elevated*	182/646 (28.2%)	268/683 (39.2%)		
Cigarette smoking				
Never regular	406/2594 (15.7%)	531/2580 (20.6%)		0.45
Ex-cigarette	1298/6229 (20.8%)	1638/6220 (26.3%)		
Current	329/1446 (22.8%)	416/1467 (28.4%)		
Treated hypertension				
Yes	942/4211 (22.4%)	1195/4246 (28.1%)		0.00
No	1091/6058 (18.0%)	1390/6021 (23.1%)		
Aspirin				
Yes	1370/6482 (21.1%)	1784/6502 (27.4%)		1.35
No	663/3787 (17.5%)	801/3765 (21.3%)		
β-blockers				
Yes	519/2661 (19.5%)	705/2618 (26.9%)		3.27
No	1514/7608 (19.9%)	1880/7649 (24.6%)		
Angiotensin-converting enzyme inhibitors				
Yes	495/1989 (24.9%)	568/1990 (28.5%)		3.75
No	1538/8280 (18.6%)	2017/8277 (24.4%)		
Vitamin allocation				
Vitamins	1014/5135 (19.7%)	1292/5134 (25.2%)		0.03
Placebo	1019/5134 (19.8%)	1293/5133 (25.2%)		
All patients	**2033/10 269 (19.8%)**	**2585/10 267 (25.2%)**		0.76 (0.72–0.81) $p < 0.0001$

0.4 0.6 0.8 1.0 1.2 1.4

Simvastatin better   Placebo better

Figure 8.17 Beneficial effects of simvaststin 40 mg across multiple subgroups of patients in the Heart Protection Study. From reference 24, with permission

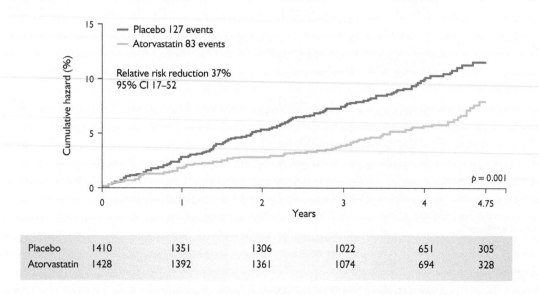

Placebo	1410	1351	1306	1022	651	305
Atorvastatin	1428	1392	1361	1074	694	328

Figure 8.18 Effect of atorvastatin in the CARDS trial on the primary end point: acute coronary syndrome, coronary revascularization, or stroke. From reference 25, with permission

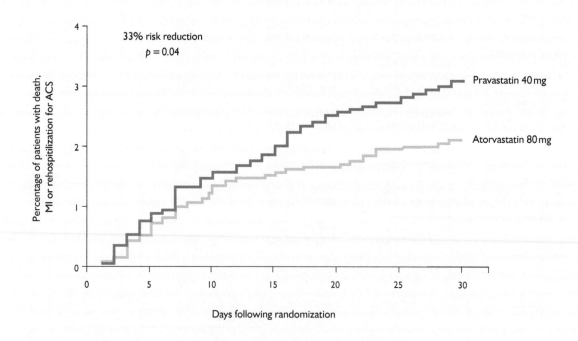

Figure 8.19 Early benefit in reducing the incidence of death, myocardial infarction or recurrent severe ischemia with intensive (high-dose) statin therapy compared with standard therapy (pravastatin 40 mg daily) in the PROVE IT-TIMI 22 trial. From reference 26, with permission

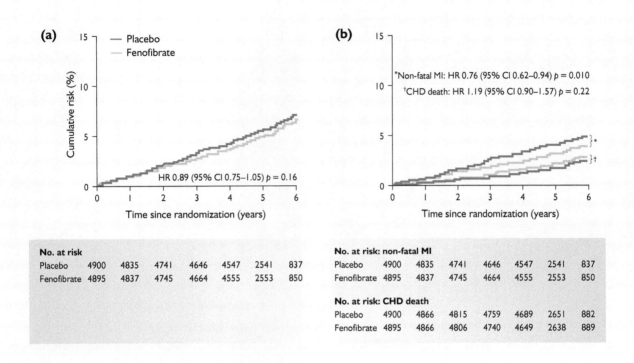

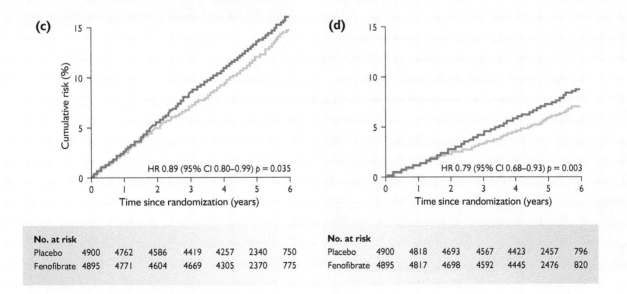

Figure 8.20 Benefit of intensive fibrate therapy in the FIELD trial. Cumulative risk to time of first coronary heart disease (CHD) events (non-fatal myocardial infarction (MI) plus CHD death (a), non-fatal MI and CHD death (b), total cardiovascular disease events (c), and coronary revascularization (d)). From reference 28, with permission

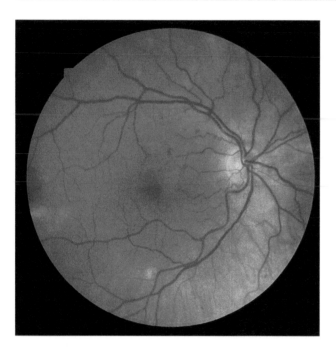

Figure 8.21 Background diabetic retinopathy with occasional scattered microaneurysms and dot hemorrhages. From reference 29, with permission

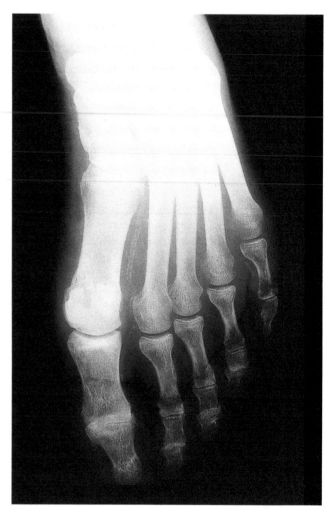

Figure 8.23 Digital arterial calcification in a diabetic foot. Peripheral vascular disease is a particularly common vascular complication of diabetes and about half of all lower limb amputations involve diabetic patients. From reference 29, with permission

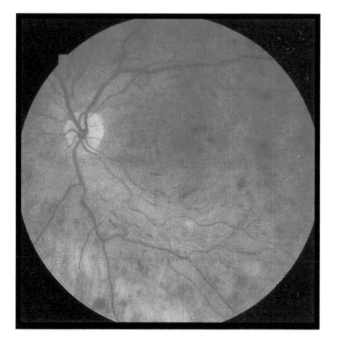

Figure 8.22 Severe background diabetic retinopathy includes venous changes, clusters and large blot hemorrhages, intraretinal microvascular abnormalities (IRMA), an early cottonwool spot and a generally ischemic appearance, This type of retinopathy is usually a prelude to proliferative change. From reference 29, with permission

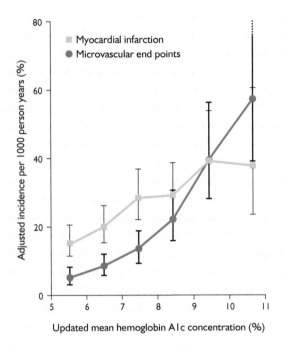

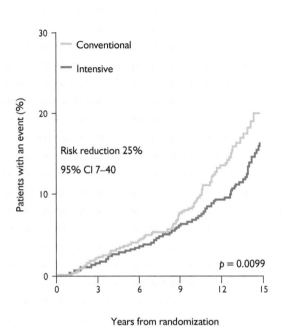

Figure 8.24 Incidence rates of myocardial infarction and microvascular end points by mean hemoglobin A1c concentration. From reference 30, with permission

Figure 8.25 Incidence rates of microvascular end points (renal failure or death, vitreous hemorrhage or photocoagulation) over time from randomization. From reference 31, with permission

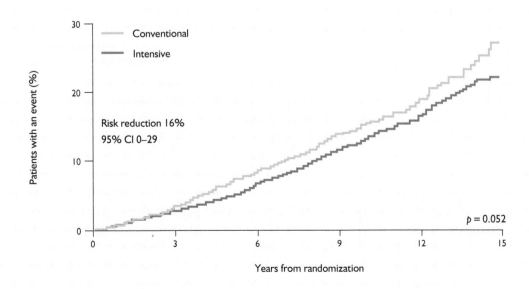

Figure 8.26 Incidence rates of myocardial infarction over time from randomization. From reference 31, with permission

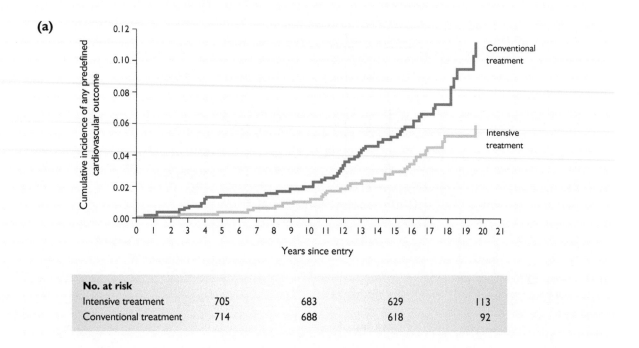

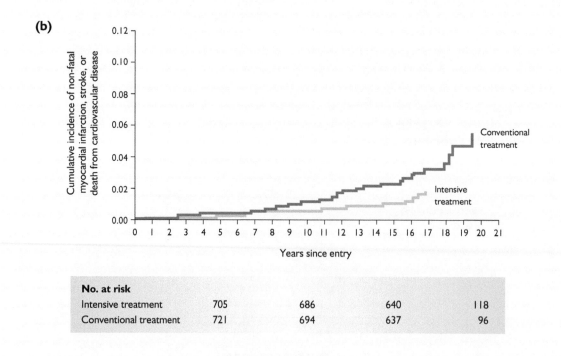

Figure 8.27 Benefit of treatment of diabetes. Cumulative incidence of the first of any predefined cardiovascular disease outcome (a) and of the first occurrence of non-fatal myocardial infarction, stroke, or death from cardiovascular disease (b). From reference 32, with permission

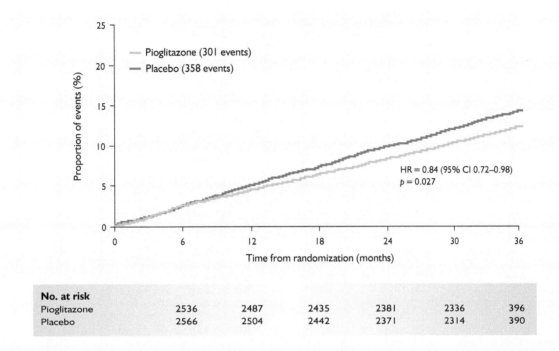

Figure 8.28 Effect of pioglitazone on a secondary end point of death, myocardial infarction or stroke. From reference 33, with permission

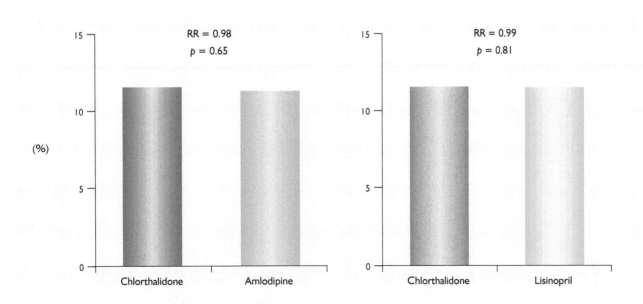

Figure 8.29 Mortality with difference antihypertensive agents in the ALLHAT trial. From reference 37, with permission

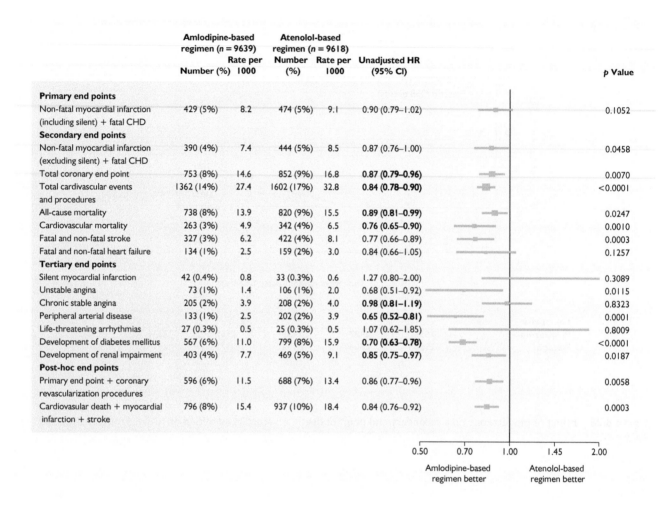

	Amlodipine-based regimen (n = 9639)		Atenolol-based regimen (n = 9618)				
	Number (%)	Rate per 1000	Number (%)	Rate per 1000	Unadjusted HR (95% CI)		p Value
Primary end points							
Non-fatal myocardial infarction (including silent) + fatal CHD	429 (5%)	8.2	474 (5%)	9.1	0.90 (0.79–1.02)		0.1052
Secondary end points							
Non-fatal myocardial infarction (excluding silent) + fatal CHD	390 (4%)	7.4	444 (5%)	8.5	0.87 (0.76–1.00)		0.0458
Total coronary end point	753 (8%)	14.6	852 (9%)	16.8	**0.87 (0.79–0.96)**		0.0070
Total cardiovascular events and procedures	1362 (14%)	27.4	1602 (17%)	32.8	**0.84 (0.78–0.90)**		<0.0001
All-cause mortality	738 (8%)	13.9	820 (9%)	15.5	**0.89 (0.81–0.99)**		0.0247
Cardiovascular mortality	263 (3%)	4.9	342 (4%)	6.5	**0.76 (0.65–0.90)**		0.0010
Fatal and non-fatal stroke	327 (3%)	6.2	422 (4%)	8.1	0.77 (0.66–0.89)		0.0003
Fatal and non-fatal heart failure	134 (1%)	2.5	159 (2%)	3.0	0.84 (0.66–1.05)		0.1257
Tertiary end points							
Silent myocardial infarction	42 (0.4%)	0.8	33 (0.3%)	0.6	1.27 (0.80–2.00)		0.3089
Unstable angina	73 (1%)	1.4	106 (1%)	2.0	0.68 (0.51–0.92)		0.0115
Chronic stable angina	205 (2%)	3.9	208 (2%)	4.0	0.98 (0.81–1.19)		0.8323
Peripheral arterial disease	133 (1%)	2.5	202 (2%)	3.9	**0.65 (0.52–0.81)**		0.0001
Life-threatening arrhythmias	27 (0.3%)	0.5	25 (0.3%)	0.5	1.07 (0.62–1.85)		0.8009
Development of diabetes mellitus	567 (6%)	11.0	799 (8%)	15.9	**0.70 (0.63–0.78)**		<0.0001
Development of renal impairment	403 (4%)	7.7	469 (5%)	9.1	**0.85 (0.75–0.97)**		0.0187
Post-hoc end points							
Primary end point + coronary revascularization procedures	596 (6%)	11.5	688 (7%)	13.4	0.86 (0.77–0.96)		0.0058
Cardiovasular death + myocardial infarction + stroke	796 (8%)	15.4	937 (10%)	18.4	0.84 (0.76–0.92)		0.0003

Figure 8.30 Benefit of amlodipine-based antihypertensive treatment compared with atenolol-based treatment. From reference 38, with permission

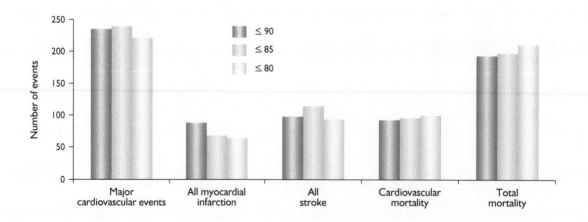

Figure 8.31 Cardiovascular events in groups based on the target blood pressure in the HOT trial. From reference 39, with permission

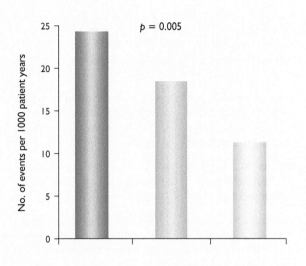

Target diastolic BP (mmHg)	Achieved systolic BP	Achieved diastolic BP	No. of patients with diabetes
≤ 90	143.7	85.2	501
≤ 85	141.4	83.2	501
≤ 80	139.7	81.1	499

Figure 8.32 Outcomes of the HOT trial of different blood pressure agents in diabetic patients. From reference 39, with permission

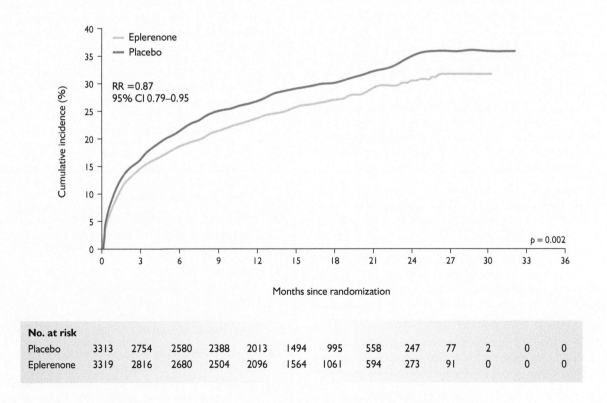

Figure 8.33 Benefits of eplerenone post myocardial infarction. Kaplan–Meier estimates of the rate of death from cardiovascular causes or hospitalization for cardiovascular events. From reference 40, with permission

REFERENCES

1. Sacks FM, Svetkey LP, Vollmer WM, et al. Effects on blood pressure of reduced dietary sodium and the Dietary Approaches to Stop Hypertension (DASH) diet. DASH-Sodium Collaborative Research Group. N Engl J Med 2001; 344: 3–10

2. Appel LJ, Sacks FM, Carey VJ, et al. Effects of protein, menosaturated fat, and carbohydrate intake on blood pressure and serum lipids: results of the OmniHeart randomized trial. JAMA 2005; 294: 2455–65

3. Willett WC. Eat, Drink and be Healthy: The Harvard Medical School Guide to Healthy Eating. New York: Simon and Schuster, 2001

4. Dansinger ML, Gleason JA, Griffith JL, et al. Comparison of the Atkins, Ornish, Weight Watchers, and Zone diets for weight loss and heart disease risk reduction: a randomized trial. JAMA 2005; 293: 43–53

5. Howard BV, Van Horn L, Hsia J, et al. Low-fat dietary pattern and risk of cardiovascular disease: the Women's Health Initiative Randomized Controlled Dietary Modification Trial. JAMA 2006; 295: 655–66

6. Manson JE, Skerret PJ, Greenland P, VanItallie TB. The escalating pandemics of obesity and sedentary lifestyle. A call to action for clinicians. Arch Intern Med 2004; 164: 249–58

7. Wirth A, Krause J. Long-term weight loss with sibutramine: a randomized controlled trial. JAMA 2001; 286: 1331–9

8. Van Gaal LF, Rissanen AM, Scheen AJ, et al. Effects of the cannabinoid-1 receptor blocker rimonabant on weight reduction and cardiovascular risk factors in overweight patients: 1-year experience from the RIO-Europe study. Lancet 2005; 365: 1389–97

9. Despres JP, Golay A, Sjostrom L. Rimonabant in Obesity-Lipids Study. Effects of rimonabant on metabolic risk factors in overweight patients with dyslipidemia. N Engl J Med 2005; 353: 2121–34

10. Pi-Sunyer FX, Aronne LJ, Heshmati HM, et al. Effect of rimonabant, a cannabinoid-1 receptor blocker, on weight and cardiometabolic risk factors in overweight or obese patients: RIO-North America: a randomized controlled trial. JAMA 2006; 295: 761–75

11. Critchley JA, Capewell S. Mortality risk reduction associated with smoking cessation in patients with coronary heart disease: a systemic review. JAMA 2003; 290: 86–97

12. Tonstad S, et al. American Heart Association Scientific Sessions 2005, Dallas, TX, November 2005

13. Hayden M, Pignone M, Phillips C, Mulrow C. Aspirin for the primary prevention of cardiovascular events: a summary of the evidence for the US Preventive Services Task Force. Ann Intern Med 2002; 236: 161–72

14. Antithrombotic Trialists' Collaboration. Collaborative meta-analysis of randomised trials of antiplatelet therapy for prevention of death, myocardial infarction, and stroke in high risk patients. BMJ 2002; 324: 71–86

15. Klint CR, Knatterud GL, Stamler J, Meier P. Persantine-Aspirin Reinfarction Study. Part II. Secondary coronary prevention with persantine and asirin. J Am Coll Cardiol 1986; 7: 251–69

16. Peters RJ, Mehta SR, Fox KA, et al. Clopidogrel in Unstable angina to prevent Recurrent Events (CURE) study. Circulation 2003; 108: 1682–7

17. CAPRIE Steering Committee. A randomised, blind, trial of clopidogrel versus aspirin in patients at risk of ischaemic events (CAPRIE). Lancet 1966; 348: 1329–39

18. Yusuf S, Mehta SR, Zhao F, et al. Clopidogrel in Unstable angina to prevent Recurrent Events Trial Investigators. Early and late effects of clopidogrel in patients with acute coronary syndromes. Circulation 2003; 107: 966–72

19. Sabatine MS, Cannon CP, Gibson CM, et al.; CLARI-TY-TIMI 28 Investigators. Addition of clopidogrel to aspirin and fibrinolytic therapy for myocardial infarction with ST-segment elevation. N Engl J Med 2005; 352: 1179–89

20. Chen ZM, Jiang LX, Chen YP; COMMIT (ClOpidogrel and Metoprolol in Myocardial Infarction Trial). Addition of clopidogrel to aspirin 45 852 patients with acute myocardial infarction: randomised placebo-controlled trial. Lancet 2005; 366: 1607–21

21. Bhatt DL, Fox KAA, Hacke W, et al.; CHARISMA Investigators. Clopidogrel and aspirin versus aspirin alone for the prevention of atherothrombotic events. N Engl J Med 2006; 354: epub

22. Schaar JA, van der Steen AF, Mastik F, et al. Intravascular palpography for vulnerable plaque assessment. J Am Coll Cardiol 2006; 47 (Suppl 8): C86–91

23. Baigent C, Keech A, Kearney PM, et al.; Cholesterol Treatment Trialists' (CCT) Collaborators. Efficacy and safety of cholesterol-lowering treatment: prospective meta-analysis of data from 90 056 participants in 14 randomised trials of statins. Lancet 2005; 366: 1267–78

24. Heart Protection Study Collaborative Group. MRC/BHF Heart Protection Study of cholesterol lowering with simvastatin in 20 536 high-risk individuals: a randomised placebo-controlled trial. Lancet 2002; 360: 7–22

25. Colhoun HM, Betteridge DJ, Durrington PN, et al.; CARDS Investigators. Primary prevention of cardiovas-

cular disease with atorvastatin in type 2 diabetes in the Collaborative Atorvastatin Diabetes Study (CARDS): multicentre randomised placebo-controlled trial. Lancet 2004; 364: 685–96

26. Ray KK, Cannon CP, McCabe CH, et al., PROVE IT-TIMI 22 Investigators. Early and late benefits of high-dose atorvastatin in patients with acute coronary syndromes: results from the PROVE IT-TIMI 22 trial. J Am Coll Cardiol 2005; 46: 1405–10

27. Cannon CP, Braunwald E, McCabe CH, et al.; Pravastatin or Atorvastatin Evaluation and Infection Therapy – Thrombolysis in Myocardial Infarction 22 Investigators. Intensive versus moderate lipid lowering with statins after acute coronary syndromes. N Engl J Med 2004; 350: 1495–504

28. Rubins HB, Robins SJ, Collins D, et al. Gemfibrozil for the secondary prevention of coronary heart disease in men with low levels of high-density lipopotein cholesterol. Veterans Affairs High Density Lipoprotein Cholesterol Intervention Trial Study Group. N Engl J Med 1999; 341: 410–18

29. Keech A, Simes RJ, Barter P, et al.; FIELD study investigators. Effects of long-term fenofibrate therapy on cardiovascular events 9795 people with type 2 diabetes mellitus (the FIELD study): randomized controlled trial. Lancet 2005; 366: 1849–61

30. Scobie IN. An Atlas of Diabetes Mellitus, 2nd edn. London: Parthenon Publishing, 2002

31. Stratton IM, Alder AI, Neil HA, et al. Association of glycaemia with macrovascular and microvascular complications of type 2 diabetes (UKPDS 35): prospective observational study. BMJ 2000; 321: 405–12

32. Nathan DM, Cleaey PA, Backlund JY, et al.; Diabetes Control and Complications Trial/Epidemiology of Diabetes Interventions and Complications (DCCT/ EDIC) Study Research Group. Intensive diabetes treatment and cardiovascular disease in patients with type 1 diabetes. N Engl J Med 2005; 353: 2643–53

33. Dormandy JA, Charbonnel B, Eckland DJ, et al.; PROactive investigators. Secondary prevention of macrovascular events in patients with type 2 diabetes in the PROactive Study (PROspective pioglitAzone Clinical Trial In macroVascular Events): a randomised controlled trial. Lancet 2005; 366: 1279–89

34. Pfutzner A, Marx N, Lubben G, et al. Improvement of cardiovascular risk markers by pioglitazone is independent from glycemic control: results from the pioneer study. J Am Coll Cardiol 2005; 45: 1925–31

35. Haffner SM, Greenberg AS, Weston WM, et al. Effect of rosiglitazone treatment on nontraditional markers of cardiovascular disease in patients with type 2 diabetes mellitus. Circulation 2002; 106: 679–84

36. Effects of treatment on morbidity in hypertension. Results in patients with diastolic blood pressures averaging 115 through 129 mmHg. JAMA 1967; 202: 1028–34

37. ALLHAT Officers and Coordinators for the ALLHAT Collaborative Research Group. The Antihypertensive and Lipid-Lowering Treatment to Prevent Heart Attack Trial. Major outcomes in high-risk hypertensive patients randomized to angiotensin-converting enzyme inhibitor of calcium channel blocker vs diuretic: The Antihypertensive and Lipid-Lowering Treatment to Prevent Heart Attack Trial (ALLHAT). JAMA 2002; 288: 2981–97

38. Dahlof B, Sever PS, Poulter NR, et al.; ASCOT Investigators. Prevention of cardiovascular events with an anti-hypertensive regimen of amlodipine adding perindopril as required versus atenolol adding bendroflumethiazide as required, in the Anglo-Scandinavian Cardiac Outcomes Trial-Blood Pressure Lowering Arm (ASCOT-BPLA): a multicentre randomised controlled trial. Lancet 2005; 366: 895–906

39. Hansson L, Zanchetti A, Carruthers SG, et al. Effects of intensive blood-pressure lowering and low-dose aspirin in patients with hypertension: principal results of the Hypertension Optimal Treatment (HOT) randomised trial. HOT Study Group. Lancet 1998; 351: 1755–62

40. Pitt B, Remme W, Zannad F, et al.; Eplerenone Post-Acute Myocardial Infarction Heart Failure Efficacy and Survival Study Investigators. Eplennone, a selective aldosterone blocker, in patients with left ventricular dysfunction after myocardial infarction. N Engl J Med 2003; 348: 1309

Index

Page numbers in *italics* refer to illustrations or tables